Drug Calculations Simplified
A Student's Guide

First Edition

Seth A. Jobson

Drug Calculations Simplified, A Student's Guide, First Edition

ISBN 978-0615820026
ISBN   0615820026

The information contained in this book is designed to help students learn how to perform various drug calculations. Recognizing the authority of individual institutions to set their own policies regarding procedures for the use of prescription medications, including calculating drug doses, this book does not supersede any institution's, public or private, right to require its health care professionals to adhere to its own policies and/or governmental, non-governmental, and quasi-governmental standards for calculating drug doses. The examples in this book are accurate as of the date of printing. However, in health care, new data constantly supplants old data, including information regarding drug doses. Accordingly, students should consult a drug guide that is updated at least monthly to ensure they have the most current data regarding drug doses.

CONTENTS

Preface

Many drug calculations are solved in exactly the same manner that most people determine that if they have eight quarters then they have two dollars. Whether realizing it or not, converting eight quarters to two dollars requires using ratios and a proportion. The vast majority of drug calculations are solved with ratios and proportions in the same manner that you convert eight quarters to two dollars. If you are anxious about math, do not worry, if you can comprehend that four quarters equals one dollar and eight quarters equals two dollars, by way of proportion, then you can perform drug calculations. If you struggle with math, in the beginning, you may have to be more formalistic about setting up proportions and solving for the unknown - the dose - but, overtime, dosing questions should become second nature, just like converting 8 quarters to two dollars. This book provides detailed answers to practice questions so that students may comprehend and memorize the entire procedure to calculating drug doses before resorting to quicker procedures.

Seth A. Jobson

Chapter 1

Prescriptions and Medication Orders
Metric System
Apothecary System

WHAT YOU SHOULD LEARN

- Prescriptions
- Medication Orders
- Metric System
- Apothecary System
- Avoirdupois system
- Converting between the various measurement systems

PRESCRIPTIONS AND MEDICATION ORDERS

Calculating drug doses is the same for both *medication orders* and prescriptions. *Medication orders* are written for patients in hospitals, nursing homes, and other types of care-settings. Prescriptions are written for ambulatory patients who can take them to retail pharmacies. Both prescriptions and medication orders contain, in brief, the date, patient's name, drug name, drug strength, dose of medication, directions, doctor's signature, or other clinician's signature. Medication orders also have the time of day that the order was written and also have information regarding the patient's specific location within a hospital or other facility. A *Medication Administration Record* (MAR) collects all of the different medication orders that a patient has. The MAR records drug names, drug strength, doses, directions, initial order date, expiration date of medication order, dates and times of administration, the site of administration, and the name of the nurse who administered the medication. In general, information relevant to drug calculations includes:

- **Drug name**: This could be the brand name or the generic name. In hospitals and institutions, there is a tendency to write drug names as generic names even when a generic version of the drug is NOT produced. Many drug names look alike when written by hand and even when printed by computer - you must carefully read the drug name. Many mistakes occur because people rush when reading drug names.

- **Drug strength**: The strength is the quantity of drug per tablet or capsule. The strength of injectable drugs is specified in terms of concentration or percents. The strength of topical drugs, such as lotions and suspensions, is usually expressed in terms of percents. Many drugs have multiple strengths. For example, atorvastatin is available in 5 mg, 10 mg, 20 mg, 40 mg, and 80 mg tablets. Lidocaine injection is available in 0.5%, 1%, 2%, and 4% solutions.

- **Dose**: The dose is the actual quantity of drug that the physician wants the patient to receive. Physicians usually write the dose in terms of mass, which is to say milligrams or grams. This includes not only orally administered tablets and capsules, but also injectable drugs. For topical drugs, such as creams and ointments, doses may be referred to as "a small amount," "a pea-sized amount," "a pearl sized amount," and "apply sparingly," among other possibilities. For topical solutions and suspensions, physicians usually instruct patients to use a small amount or sufficient amount to cover a certain area. For oral drugs that are liquids, doses may be written in terms of volume or milligrams or grams or both. There are not any hard and fast legal rules that doctors and other prescribers must follow when writing a dose, just generally accepted conventions that one must learn through hands-on experience.

- **Dosage form**: Dosage forms include tablets, capsules, creams, ointments, oral suspensions, oral solutions, topical suspensions, topical solutions, and injections. The dosage form influences the quantity of medication to be dispensed to a patient.

- **Route of administration**: These include oral, sublingual, intranasal, inhalation, topical, rectal, intravaginally, opthalmic, otic (ears), intramuscular, subcutaneous, intravenous, intra-arterial, and intrathecal.

- **Frequency**: Oral drugs are usually dosed one, two, three, or four times daily; some oral drugs, such as acyclovir, can be dosed five times daily. Injectable drugs are generally dosed every 4, 6, 8, 12, or 24 hours.

- **Start and Stop dates**: For prescriptions, the start and stop dates depend on when the patient has the prescription filled. For medication order in hospitals and other institutions, start dates are controlled by when a physician writes an order. Stop dates depend on a combination of physician instructions and a particular hospital or institutions policies on when medications should be stopped.

MEASUREMENT SYSTEMS

Before being able to calculate drug doses or other drug calculations, you must understand the different measurement systems. In healthcare, three different measurement systems are used, the Metric System, Apothecary System, and Avoirdupois system. All three are commonly used. You should be familiar with the basics of each.

METRIC SYSTEM

The metric system (also called the International System of Units) recognizes units for mass, volume, and length. The unit of mass is the kilogram. The unit of volume is the liter. The unit of length is the meter.

The definition of a kilogram has changed over the years. Presently, a kilogram is officially the amount of mass in a certain piece of platinum-iridium cylinder kept at Sèvres, France. Originally, a kilogram was defined as the mass of a liter of water. A kilogram and liter of water have the same mass. For visualization purposes, a liter of water is about 5% larger than a quart of milk.

A gram is presently defined as 1/1000 of this certain piece of platinum-iridium cylinder. Originally, a gram was defined as the mass of a cubic centimeter (1 cc) of water at 4^0 C. This amounts to about 1/5 of the amount of water in a teaspoon; yes, teaspoons vary in size, this is just to give you something to picture.

1 kilogram(kg) = 1000 grams (g)
1 gram = 1000 milligrams (mg)
1 milligram = 1000 micrograms (mcg)

1 kilogram = 1000 grams = 1,000,000 milligrams

The liter is the basic unit of volume in the metric system. In health care practice, you will generally be working with milliliters, but some IVs are measured in liters (L). A liter is the volume of a cube whose sides are 10 centimeters long.

Here is a brief review of the relationships of volume in the metric system.

1 liter (L) = 1000 milliliters
1 ml = 1000 microliters (ul)
1 ml = 1 cc

1 Liter = 1000 milliliters

Converting From One Metric Unit to Another

The Metric System's advantage over other systems is that everything is based on powers of ten - so you can do the math in your head. Basing everything on powers of ten avoids the need of setting up proportions and solving them when converting from one unit to the next. Rather, you just have to move the decimal point, to the left or right, a certain number of places, depending on the specific change in units that you want to accomplish.

For example, when changing from grams to milligrams, you are moving from a big unit to a small unit - it takes more small units to equal a larger unit - therefore, move the decimal point to the right so the number becomes bigger to compensate for the unit becoming smaller. You need many more small pieces to equal one large piece. One gram has been arbitrarily declared to equal 1000 milligrams. So when changing from grams to milligrams you move the decimal point three places (a factor of a thousand (a power of ten)) to the right.

Here is another way to think about converting from grams to milli-grams:

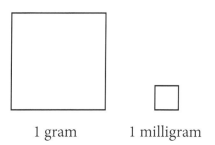

1 gram   1 milligram

The milligram unit is smaller than the gram unit. Suppose we call the larger square above 1 gram and the smaller square 1 milligram. From the picture, you could cut the 1 gram square up into many small-er 1 milligram squares. So when converting from grams to milligrams, the number ("1" here) becomes larger while the unit becomes smaller. This holds true any time you convert from a larger unit to a smaller unit - the number becomes larger.

And, the converse is true, when you convert from a small unit to a larger unit, the number becomes smaller. You only need a fraction of the 1 gram square to cover the same area covered by the 1 mg square. So when converting from milligrams to grams, the number becomes smaller, while the unit becomes larger. No, grams and milligrams are not geometric squares, this is just a visual aid.

Remember, that the number and unit always move in opposite directions when converting from one unit to another in the metric system.

Example Practice Problem:

Convert 2 grams to milligrams.

Answer: First recognize that there actually is an implied decimal point after the "2" - it is just simply almost never written. You can rewrite the "2" as "2.0". A brief digression, in health care, you NEVER actu-ally write the decimal point and zero after a 1, 2, 3, 4, 5, 6, 7, 8, or 9 because this can lead to a ten-fold overdose if someone does not see the decimal point and reads the number as a "10" or "20" etc. In these practice problems, you can write the decimal point if it helps you. Since 1 gram equals 1000 milligrams, you multiply the number of grams (2) by 1000, which is the same as adding three zeros to the right of the decimal point. The 2 is a single digit, so add three zeros after it to get 2000, the answer.

Example Practice Problem:

Convert 0.3 grams to milligrams.

Answer: Since each 1 gram equals 1000 milligrams, multiply the number of grams (0.3) by 1000, which is the same as moving the decimal point three places to the right, which gives the answer of 300 mg.

APOTHECARY SYSTEM

The apothecary system has units of measure for both volume and mass. The apothecary system's units of measure for volume are commonly used, today. In contrast, the apothecary system's units of measure for mass are rarely used. In the apothecary system, volumes of measure include fluid ounces, pints, quarts, and gallons. The relationship between these units of measure is as follows:

16 fluidounces = 1 pint
2 pints = 1 quart
4 quarts = 1 gallon
1 fluid ounce = 29.57 ml exactly
1 fluid ounce = 30 ml approximately

The "fluid ounce" is the basic unit of measure that you will see in health care. A fluid ounce equals exactly 29.57 ml - however, you will predominantly see a fluid ounce as being 30 ml. It is abbreviated as "oz." or sometimes you will see "fl. oz." As a practical matter, you will be able to deduce that if the doctor is writing for a cough syrup and writes "4 oz," you know that he or she is referring to the fluid ounce and not the weight ounce because the prescription is for a syrup which is measured as a liquid.

The apothecary system uses "grains" (gr) as its main unit of measure for mass. 480 grains equals one ounce. 12 ounces equals one pound. And, 5760 grains equals one pound.

480 grains = 1 ounce
12 ounces = 1 pound
5760 grains = 1 pound

AVOIRDUPOIS SYSTEM

The avoirdupois system recognizes units of measure for mass. The three units are grains (gr), ounces (oz), and pounds. 437.5 grains equal one ounce. 16 ounces equal one pound. Here, 7000 grains equals one pound. This last unit is the unit used in the United States for comparing ounces to pounds. (The Apothecaries system also has "ounces" and "pounds"; in that system 12 ounces equals one pound.)

16 ounces = 1 pound
1 ounce = 30 grams (approximately, also most commonly used)
1 ounce = 28.35 grams (exactly, less commonly used)

CONVERTING UNITS BETWEEN THE VARIOUS SYSTEMS

The following chart provides a comprehensive list of the conversions that you should know:

CONVERTING MASS

1 pound (avoirdupois) = 0.454 kg
1 kilogram = 2.20 pounds (avoirdupois)
1 ounce (avoirdupois) = 28.35 grams exactly (least used)
1 ounce = 30 grams approximately (most commonly used)
1 pound (avoirdupois) = 454 grams exactly
1 pound (avoirdupois) = 480 grams approximately
1 grain = 65 mg

CONVERTING VOLUME

1 teaspoonful = 5 ml
1 tablespoon = 15 ml
1 fluid ounce = 29.57 ml exactly (least used)
1 fluid ounce = 30 ml approximately (most commonly used)
1 pint = 473 ml
1 pint = 16 ounces
1 U.S. gallon = 3785 ml

Mastery of this list will allow you to pass your exams and work competently.

Review

Prescriptions and medication orders provide detailed information, allowing other health care workers to provide medications to patients. Medication orders are used in hospitals, nursing homes, and other types of care facilities. Medication orders have several important pieces of information: the date and time written, patient's name, patient's identification number, room number, drug name, drug strength, dose, and directions. Throughout the day, medication orders are transferred to a patient's medication administration record. The medication administration record records all of the different medications that a patient has received or is receiving.

Physicians and other clinicians can write prescriptions and medication orders using the Metric System, Apothecary System, or Avoirdupois System. You must know: 1) the basics units of each system 2) how to convert from one unit to another unit in the same system, and 3) how to convert units from one system to another system. Many computer systems are programmed just to use the metric system. In health care, you will mainly use the kilogram (kg), gram (g), and milligram (mg) when dealing with mass. For volume, you will use the liter (L) and milliliter (ml). The meter is also used to measure body surface area, which is discussed in chapter 8.

Practice Problems:

1. Convert 5 grams to milligrams.
2. Convert 0.5 grams to milligrams.
3. Convert 4 grams to milligrams.
4. Convert 0.4 grams to milligrams.
5. Convert 70 grams to milligrams.
6. Convert 1500 milligrams to grams.
7. Convert 2000 milligrams to grams.
8. Convert 3000 milligrams to grams.
9. Convert 100 milligrams to grams.
10. Convert 50 milligrams to grams.
11. Convert 2 teaspoons to milliliters.
12. Approximately, 2 fluid ounces equals how many ml?
13. Convert 2 grains to milligrams.
14. Convert 220 pounds to kilograms.
15. Convert 50 kilograms to pounds.
16. Convert 2 tablespoons to ml.
17. Convert 30 ml to teaspoons.
18. Convert 2 ounces to grams approximately.
19. Convert 2 quarts to gallons.
20. Convert 10 ml to teaspoons.

Answers:

1. Multiplying by 1000 equals 5000 milligrams.
2. Multiplying by 1000 equals 500 milligrams.
3. Multiplying by 1000 equals 4000 milligrams.
4. Multiplying by 1000 equals 400 milligrams.
5. Multiplying by 1000 equals 70,000 milligrams.
6. Dividing by 1000 equals 1.5 grams.
7. Dividing by 1000 equals 2 grams.
8. Dividing by 1000 equals 3 grams.

9.   Dividing by 1000 equals 0.1 grams.

10.   Dividing by 1000 equals 0.05 grams.

11.   1 teaspoon equals 5 ml. 2 teaspoons equals 10 ml.

12.   1 fluid ounce approximately equals 30 ml. 2 fl. oz. equals 60 ml.

13.   1 grain equals 65 mg. 2 grains equals 130 mg.

14.   1 pound equals 0.4545 kilograms. 220 pounds equals 100 kg.

15.   1 kg equals 2.2 pounds. 50 kg equals 110 pounds.

16.   1 tablespoon equals 15 ml. 2 tbsp. equals 30 ml.

17.   5 ml equals 1 tsp. 30 ml equals 6 tsp.

18.   1 ounce equals approximately 30 g. 2 oz. equals 60 g.

19.   4 quarts equals 1 gallon. 2 quarts equals 0.5 gallons.

20.   5 ml equals 1 teaspoon. 10 ml equals 2 teaspoon.

Chapter 2

Dose Calculations

What you should learn:

- Several ways to solve pharmaceutical calculations
- Using proportions to calculate what quantity to give
- Understand ratios
- Understand proportions

Introduction:
Several Ways to Solve Dose Calculations

Drug dosing questions can be solved with proportions. You can setup a proportion several different ways, which are discussed throughout this chapter. You should note, though, that these "different" ways are just slight variations of each other. Despite the flexibility in setting up proportions, there are incorrect ways of setting up proportions and these incorrect ways are noted below.

Why the need for a proportion? To calculate the volume of drug to give to a patient. Doctors write many drug doses in terms of mass (milligrams or grams). When the medication order is for a liquid drug, such as an injectable drug, you need to calculate the VOLUME (milliliters) of drug that contains the dose prescribed and use a syringe to withdraw that amount. A proportion between the concentration of the drug in the manufacturer's stock vial on the left side of the equals sign and the volume and dose of drug on the right side of the equals sign allows you to solve for the volume of drug needed.

$$\frac{mg}{ml} = \frac{Dose\ in\ mg}{Volume\ in\ ml\ you\ need\ to\ withdraw\ from\ vial}$$

The above equation, as written, is not in the simplest to use format. You can rearrange this equation to make calculating the volume much easier. The simplest to use version of the above equation is:

$$\text{Volume needed} = \frac{\text{Dose}}{\text{Drug Concentration}}$$

Because the drug concentration is a fraction the above equation can be rewritten as:

$$\text{Volume needed} = \text{Dose} \times \frac{\text{ml}}{\text{mg}}$$

Here, the "ml/mg" is simply the reciprocal of the drug concentration.

If the drug concentration is stated in milligrams per 1 ml, then you simply have to divide the dose by the drug concentration. If the drug concentration is in anything other than milligrams per 1 ml, then you have to either: 1) convert the concentration to milligrams per 1 ml or 2) use the equation that is immediately above. For example if the concentration was 10 mg/2ml, you can convert that to 5 mg/1ml or divide the dose by 10 mg and then remember to multiply by 2 ml to get the right answer. Of course, the units do not have to be mg. The units could be grams or micrograms, etc.

A Brief Note about Drug Concentrations

Injectable drugs, as liquids, are manufactured with certain concentrations: this means that there is a certain MASS quantity of drug per a certain VOLUME quantity of solution or suspension. Injectable drugs come in many different types of concentrations including:

A) $\dfrac{10\ \text{mg}}{1\ \text{ml}}$ B) $\dfrac{10\ \text{mg}}{2\ \text{ml}}$ C) $\dfrac{20\ \text{mg}}{1\ \text{ml}}$ D) $\dfrac{20\ \text{mg}}{2\ \text{ml}}$ E) $\dfrac{10\ \text{mg}}{5\ \text{ml}}$ F) $\dfrac{2\ \text{mg}}{1\ \text{ml}}$

(Yes, some of these are equivalent, but concentrations are not always written in the lowest possible terms.) Note that the denominators are not always 1ml - this is important in calculating the volume.

Using Proportions to Calculate What Quantity to Give

Method #1

Let's look at a quick example and the several different ways that you can write a proportion to calculate the volume containing the prescribed dose of drug. A doctor writes a medication order for 100 mg of drug "A" to be administered to a patient. You have a manufacturer's vial that has 10 mg per 1 ml, which is written on the label as:

$$\frac{10 \text{ mg}}{1 \text{ ml}}$$

You can read this fraction as saying, "there are 10 mg of drug per each 1 ml of solution." **As a matter of preference, because it makes calculations easier, flip the concentration and write it as:**

$$\frac{1 \text{ ml}}{10 \text{ mg}}$$

You can read this fraction as saying, "each 1 ml of solution has 10 mg of drug." Back to the original question: how many ml of solution have 100 mg of drug "A"?

Here is a simple proportion that allows you to calculate the volume of solution that contains 100 mg of drug "A":

$$\frac{1 \text{ ml}}{10 \text{ mg}} = \frac{X \text{ ml}}{100 \text{ mg}} \qquad \text{Equation \#1}$$

To make the calculation easier, the concentration is inverted to 1ml/10mg. It means that every 1 ml of solution has 10 mg of drug. The "100 mg" is the dose prescribed. You have to calculate the volume of solution that has 100 mg of drug "A". **Here, "X ml" represents the volume of solution that has 100 mg of drug "A" - this is the quantity that will be given to the patient.**

As the proportion is currently written, you should read it as saying, "in the manufacturer's stock vial, each 1 ml has 10 mg of drug, and X ml has 100 mg of drug."

One simple way of solving these problems is noting that since these two ratios are equal, by definition, whatever you do to the denominator (10 mg), you have to do to the numerator (1 ml). Here, the 10 mg was multiplied by 10 to get 100 mg. Therefore, you have to multiply the 1 ml by 10, which gives you the answer of 10 ml. Sometimes the math won't be that simple.

Alternatively, you can write out the algebraic steps needed to calculate the volume needed. Algebraically, you have to isolate X ml so you can determine its value. As a first step, you multiply both sides by "100 mg," resulting in "100 mg" now being in the numerator on the left and canceled out of the denominator on the right, as follows:

$$\frac{100 \text{ mg} \times 1 \text{ ml}}{10 \text{ mg}} = \frac{X \text{ ml}}{\cancel{100 \text{ mg}}} \times \cancel{100 \text{ mg}}$$

This simplifies to:

$$\frac{100 \text{ mg} \times 1 \text{ ml}}{10 \text{ mg}} = X \text{ ml}$$

Second, divide the 100 mg by the 10 mg. The answer is 10 without any units, that is without the "mg," as follows:

$$10 \times 1 \text{ ml} = X \text{ ml}$$

The above simplifies to the correct answer of:

$$10 \text{ ml} = X \text{ ml}$$

So, we need 10 ml of liquid drug "A" to get 100 mg of drug "A."

Method #2

In short, the simplest way to calculate a dose of an injectable drug or other liquid drug is to use the following formula:

$$\text{Volume needed} = \frac{\text{Dose Prescribed by Doctor}}{\text{Concentration of the stock vial}}$$

As a consequence of the fact that the "concentration of the stock vial" is itself a fraction, the above equation can be written as:

$$\text{Volume needed} = \frac{\text{Dose}}{\frac{\text{mg}}{\text{ml}}}$$

Dividing a number (Dose) by a fraction (the concentration) is the same as multiplying by the inverse (upside down version) of the fraction. To make the above equation easier to use and read, it is often written as follows, and you should memorize this formula:

$$\text{Volume needed} = \frac{\text{Dose}}{\text{mg}} \times \text{ml}$$

Note that most of the time the concentration of injectable drugs and oral liquids is in terms of milligrams per ml, as shown in the above equation. If the manufacturer's stock vial has the concentration stated in different terms, then use those terms, such as milliequivalents per ml. Sometimes you may see the concentration in terms of grams per so many milliliters - adjust the units in the equation accordingly.

For convenience, Equation #1 is often rewritten as:

$$\text{X ml} = \frac{100\ \text{mg}}{10\ \text{mg}} \times 1\ \text{ml} \qquad \text{Equation \#2}$$

The above equation can also be written as:

$$\text{X ml} = 100\ \text{mg} \times \frac{1\ \text{ml}}{10\ \text{mg}} \qquad \text{Equation \#3}$$

The "1 ml" represents the volume component of drug "A's" concentration and the "10 mg" represents the mass or quantity component of drug "A's" concentration. The above two equations are equivalent to Equation #1 above.

You should note that if the manufacturer's stock vial has a concentration of 10 mg/2ml then the above equation would be written as:

$$X \text{ ml} = 100 \text{ mg} \times \frac{2 \text{ ml}}{10 \text{ mg}}$$

You read the above equation as saying, "the volume needed equals the dose **multiplied** by the **inverse** of the concentration on the manufacturer's stock bottle."

General Rules for Setting up Proportions

You must follow one of two rules. First, both of your numerators (the numbers on the top of the ratios) must have the same units, either both are "ml" or both are "mg," as follows:

$$\frac{\text{ml}}{\text{mg}} = \frac{\text{ml}}{\text{mg}} \quad \text{or} \quad \frac{\text{mg}}{\text{ml}} = \frac{\text{mg}}{\text{ml}}$$

Second, both the numerator and denominator in the ratio on the left side of the equals sign must have the same units and both the numerator and denominator on the right side of the equals sign must have the same units, as follows:

$$\frac{\text{mg}}{\text{mg}} = \frac{\text{ml}}{\text{ml}} \quad \text{or} \quad \frac{\text{ml}}{\text{ml}} = \frac{\text{mg}}{\text{mg}}$$

Method #3

Some people may not feel comfortable inverting the manufacturer's drug concentration. If so, you may feel more comfortable writing the initial equation above as:

$$\frac{10 \text{ mg}}{1 \text{ ml}} = \frac{100 \text{ mg}}{X \text{ ml}}$$

and then solving for X ml. Here the proportion can be read as saying, "there are 10 mg in 1 ml and this equals 100 mg in X ml." This approach requires the additional step of multiplying both sides by "X ml," resulting in X ml now being in the numerator on the left side of the equation, as follows:

$$\frac{\text{X ml} \times 10 \text{ mg}}{1 \text{ ml}} = \frac{100 \text{ mg}}{\cancel{\text{X ml}}} \times \cancel{\text{X ml}}$$

This simplifies to:

$$\frac{\text{X ml} \times 10 \text{ mg}}{1 \text{ ml}} = 100 \text{ mg}$$

Now, you divide both sides by 10 mg, yielding:

$$\frac{\text{X ml} \times \cancel{10 \text{ mg}}}{1 \text{ ml} \times \cancel{10 \text{ mg}}} = \frac{100 \text{ mg}}{10 \text{ mg}}$$

This simplifies to:

$$\frac{\text{X ml}}{1 \text{ ml}} = \frac{100 \text{ mg}}{10 \text{ mg}}$$

Now divide the 100 mg by 10 mg, leaving you with 10 without any units, as follows:

$$\frac{\text{X ml}}{1 \text{ ml}} = 10$$

Now, multiply both sides by "1 ml," which erases it from the left side and places it on the right side next to the "10," as follows:

$$\text{X ml} = 10 \times 1 \text{ ml}$$

which simplifies to:

$$X \text{ ml} = 10 \text{ ml}$$

The correct answer is 10 ml (the same as above).

Wrong Method for Setting up Proportions

You cannot start with like units on a diagonal to each other. For example, you cannot put mg in the numerator in the ratio on the left side of the equals sign and also put mg in the denominator in the ratio on the right side of the equals sign. Additionally, you cannot put mg in the denominator in the ratio on the left side of the equals sign and also put mg in the numerator in the ratio on the right side of the equals sign. You cannot start a proportion with the following:

$$\frac{\text{ml}}{\text{mg}} = \frac{\text{mg}}{\text{ml}} \qquad \text{or} \qquad \frac{\text{mg}}{\text{ml}} = \frac{\text{ml}}{\text{mg}}$$

Otherwise, you will get an incorrect answer. For example, if you started with:

$$\frac{1 \text{ ml}}{10 \text{ mg}} = \frac{100 \text{ mg}}{X \text{ ml}} = \textbf{WRONG STARTING POINT}$$

You would get an incorrect answer.

Calculating Doses for Tablets and Capsules

If the prescription or medication order is for tablets or capsules, you just have to determine how many tablets or capsules are needed to equal the dose prescribed by the doctor. The vast majority of the time a tablet or capsule is available that exactly matches the dose prescribed. Sometimes, though, you may have to double the number of tablets or capsules to equal the dose prescribed. Example, if a medication order is for 1000 mg of a drug and the drug only comes in 500 mg tablets, then you have to give the patient two tablets at a time to equal 1000 mg, simple enough. Or, sometimes you may have to cut a tablet in half to administer the correct dose. For example, if the dose is 500 mg and the only available tablet is a 1000 mg tablet, then you need to cut the tablet in half, provided that the manufacturer states, in the package insert, that the tablet can be cut in half.

Example:

A doctor writes a prescription to dispense drug "C" 750 mg to be administered orally. Drug "C" is available as 250 mg tablets only. How many tablets does the patient need to take for each dose? If you do not immediately see the answer, then write a proportion as follows:

$$\frac{1 \text{ tablet}}{250 \text{ mg}} = \frac{X \text{ tablets}}{750 \text{ mg}}$$

Solve for X tablets by multiplying both sides by 750 mg:

$$\frac{750 \text{ mg} \times 1 \text{ tablet}}{250 \text{ mg}} = \frac{X \text{ tablets}}{750 \text{ mg}} \times 750 \text{ mg}$$

This simplifies to:

$$\frac{750 \text{ mg} \times 1 \text{ tablet}}{250 \text{ mg}} = X \text{ tablets}$$

Divide 750 mg by 250 mg, yielding:

$$3 \times 1 \text{ tablet} = X \text{ tablets}$$

Finally, $3 \text{ tablets} = X \text{ tablets}$

So, the patient needs three tablets per dose.

If you had difficulty with these examples, the remainder of this chapter, after the practice problems, reviews the basics of fractions, ratios, and proportions. Reviewing these topics should make understanding the above examples easier.

Review

You can use any of several possible starting points for calculating the volume that is needed of a liquid drug to provide the dose prescribed by a doctor. Use whichever starting point you are comfortable with. Recognize that the different starting points are all just different versions of a standard proportion.

Most of the time when you want to calculate the volume of a liquid drug, oral or injection, you simply have to divide the dose by the concentration so long a the concentration is in terms of milligrams per 1 ml. If not, you have two options: 1) convert the concentration to milligrams per 1 ml or 2) divide the dose by the mg part of the concentration and then multiply by the ml part of the concentration, if you forget to multiply by the ml part of the concentration then you will calculate a lower dose than is actually required.

Practice Problems

For each of the following questions, calculate the volume of drug (from the manufacturer's stock vial) that contains the prescribed dose of drug.

1)   A doctor prescribes 20 mg of an injectable drug that is available in a concentration of 2 mg/1ml. What volume of drug contains the prescribed dose?

2)   A doctor prescribes 30 mg of an injectable drug that is available in a concentration of 5 mg/5ml. What volume of drug contains the prescribed dose?

3)   A doctor prescribes 50 mg of an injectable drug that is available in a concentration of 25 mg/1ml. What volume of drug contains the

prescribed dose?

4)   A doctor prescribes 100 mg of an injectable drug that is available in a concentration of 20 mg/1ml. What volume of drug contains the prescribed dose?

5)   A doctor prescribes 100 mg of an injectable drug that is available in a concentration of 25 mg/1ml. What volume of drug contains the prescribed dose?

6)   A nurse practitioner prescribes 250 mg of amoxicillin to be given every 8 hours to a patient. You have a stock bottle that has 50 mg/1ml? What volume of drug contains the prescribed dose?

7)   A physician's assistant prescribes 750 mg of a drug that is available in a concentration of 15 mg/1ml. What volume of drug contains the prescribed dose?

8)   A nurse practitioner prescribes 1000 mg of a drug that is available in a concentration of 50 mg/1ml. What volume of drug contains the prescribed dose?

9)   A doctor prescribes 500 mg of a drug that is available in a concentration of 10 mg/1ml. What volume of drug contains the prescribed dose?

10)   A physician's assistant prescribes 400 mg of a drug that is available in a concentration of 80 mg/1ml. What volume of drug contains the prescribed dose?

Answers

1) One possible starting point is:

$$\frac{1 \text{ ml}}{2 \text{ mg}} = \frac{X \text{ ml}}{20 \text{ mg}}$$

Solve for X ml by multiplying both sides by 20 mg so you can isolate "X ml" by itself and determine its value, as follows:

$$\frac{20 \text{ mg} \times 1 \text{ ml}}{2 \text{ mg}} = \frac{X \text{ ml}}{20 \text{ mg}} \times 20 \text{ mg}$$

Simplifying this leaves you with:

$$\frac{20 \text{ mg} \times 1 \text{ ml}}{2 \text{ mg}} = X \text{ ml}$$

Dividing by 2 mg leaves you with:

$$10 \times 1 \text{ ml} = X \text{ ml}$$

This simplifies to:

$$10 \text{ ml} = X \text{ ml}$$

So the answer is 10 ml. All of the above problems can be solved using exactly the same procedure.

2)   Start with the following proportion:

$$\frac{5 \text{ ml}}{5 \text{ mg}} = \frac{X \text{ ml}}{30 \text{ mg}}$$

Recognize that because you have to multiply the 5 mg in the denominator by 6 to get 30 mg you then also have to multiply the 5 ml in the numerator by 6, which gives you the correct answer of 30 ml. You can also use the same steps outlined above.

3)   Start with:

$$\frac{1 \text{ ml}}{25 \text{ mg}} = \frac{X \text{ ml}}{50 \text{ mg}}$$

It should be easy to recognize that you have to multiply 25 mg by 2 to get 50 mg, so therefore you multiply the 1 ml by 2 to get 2 ml, which is the answer. Also:

$$\frac{50 \text{ mg} \times 1 \text{ ml}}{25 \text{ mg}} = \frac{X \text{ ml}}{\cancel{50 \text{ mg}}} \times \cancel{50 \text{ mg}}$$

Simplify this to:

$$2 \times 1 \text{ ml} = X \text{ ml}$$

Simplifying again leaves you with:

$$2 \text{ ml} = X \text{ ml}$$

Your answer is 2 ml.

4)   Start with the following proportion:

$$\frac{1 \text{ ml}}{20 \text{ mg}} = \frac{X \text{ ml}}{100 \text{ mg}}$$

Isolate Xml by itself so you can determine its value. Isolate it by multiplying both sides by 100 mg, which removes the 100 mg from the right side of the equation, leaving X ml alone on the left side, as follows:

$$\frac{100 \text{ mg} \times 1 \text{ ml}}{20 \text{ mg}} = \frac{X \text{ ml}}{\cancel{100 \text{ mg}}} \times \cancel{100 \text{ mg}}$$

This simplifies to:

$$\frac{100 \text{ mg} \times 1 \text{ ml}}{20 \text{ mg}} = X \text{ ml}$$

Divide 100 mg by 20 mg:

$$5 \times 1 \text{ ml} = X \text{ ml}$$

Finally,

$$5 \text{ ml} = X \text{ ml}$$

Your answer is 5 ml.

5)   Start with:

$$\frac{1 \text{ ml}}{25 \text{ mg}} = \frac{X \text{ ml}}{100 \text{ mg}}$$

Isolate X ml by multiplying both sides by 100 mg:

$$\frac{100 \text{ mg} \times 1 \text{ ml}}{25 \text{ mg}} = \frac{X \text{ ml}}{\cancel{100 \text{ mg}}} \times \cancel{100 \text{ mg}}$$

Simplify to:

$$\frac{100 \text{ mg} \times 1 \text{ ml}}{25 \text{ mg}} = X \text{ ml}$$

Divide 100 mg by 25 mg, yielding:

$$4 \times 1 \text{ ml} = X \text{ ml}$$

Simplify once more to:

$$4 \text{ ml} = X \text{ ml}$$

The answer is 4 ml.

6)   Start with:

$$\frac{1 \text{ ml}}{50 \text{ mg}} = \frac{X \text{ ml}}{250 \text{ mg}}$$

Multiply both sides by 250 mg so you can isolate X ml, as follows:

$$\frac{250 \text{ mg} \times 1 \text{ ml}}{50 \text{ mg}} = \frac{X \text{ ml}}{\cancel{250 \text{ mg}}} \times \cancel{250 \text{ mg}}$$

This simplifies to:

$$\frac{250 \text{ mg} \times 1 \text{ ml}}{50 \text{ mg}} = X \text{ ml}$$

Divide 250 mg by 50 mg:

$$5 \times 1 \text{ ml} = X \text{ ml}$$

Simplify again to:

$$5 \text{ ml} = X \text{ ml}$$

The answer is 5 ml.

7)   Start with:

$$\frac{1 \text{ ml}}{15 \text{ mg}} = \frac{X \text{ ml}}{750 \text{ mg}}$$

Multiply both sides by 750 mg:

$$\frac{750 \text{ mg} \times 1 \text{ ml}}{15 \text{ mg}} = \frac{X \text{ ml}}{\cancel{750 \text{ mg}}} \times \cancel{750 \text{ mg}}$$

Simplify to:

$$\frac{750 \text{ mg} \times 1 \text{ ml}}{15 \text{ mg}} = X \text{ ml}$$

Divide 750 mg by 15 mg:

$$50 \times 1 \text{ ml} = X \text{ ml}$$

Finally, we have:

$$50 \text{ ml} = X \text{ ml}$$

The answer is 50 ml.

8)   Start with:

$$\frac{1 \text{ ml}}{50 \text{ mg}} = \frac{X \text{ ml}}{1000 \text{ mg}}$$

Isolate X ml by multiplying both sides by 1000 mg, as follows:

$$\frac{1000 \text{ mg} \times 1 \text{ ml}}{50 \text{ mg}} = \frac{X \text{ ml}}{\cancel{1000 \text{ mg}}} \times \cancel{1000 \text{ mg}}$$

Simplify to:

$$\frac{1000 \text{ mg} \times 1 \text{ ml}}{50 \text{ mg}} = X \text{ ml}$$

Divide 1000 mg by 50 mg:

$$20 \times 1 \text{ ml} = X \text{ ml}$$

Finally, we have:

$$20 \text{ ml} = X \text{ ml}$$

The answer is 20 ml.

9)   Start with:

$$\frac{1 \text{ ml}}{10 \text{ mg}} = \frac{X \text{ ml}}{500 \text{ mg}}$$

Multiply both sides by 500 mg:

$$\frac{500 \text{ mg} \times 1 \text{ ml}}{10 \text{ mg}} = \frac{X \text{ ml}}{\cancel{500 \text{ mg}}} \times \cancel{500 \text{ mg}}$$

Simplify to:

$$\frac{500 \text{ mg} \times 1 \text{ ml}}{10 \text{ mg}} = X \text{ ml}$$

Divide 500 mg by 10 mg:

$$50 \times 1 \text{ ml} = X \text{ ml}$$

Simplify to:

$$50 \text{ ml} = X \text{ ml}$$

The answer is 50 ml.

10)   Start with:

$$\frac{1 \text{ ml}}{80 \text{ mg}} = \frac{X \text{ ml}}{400 \text{ mg}}$$

Isolate Xml as follows:

$$\frac{400 \text{ mg} \times 1 \text{ ml}}{80 \text{ mg}} = \frac{X \text{ ml}}{\cancel{400 \text{ mg}}} \times \cancel{400 \text{ mg}}$$

Simplify to:

$$\frac{400 \text{ mg} \times 1 \text{ ml}}{80 \text{ mg}} = X \text{ ml}$$

Divide 400 mg by 80 mg:

$$5 \times 1 \text{ ml} = X \text{ ml}$$

Finally, we have:

$$5 \text{ ml} = X \text{ ml}$$

The answer is 5 ml.

Ratios

Ratios tell you the relative size of two numbers. For example, "1/2" is a fraction that tells you for every 1 of something you have 2 of something else. Although you can, please don't read the fraction "1/2" as "one-half." For our purposes, read it as "for every 1 of something we have two of something else...." Ratios are written as one number over another number as follows:

$$\frac{1}{2} \quad \text{or} \quad \frac{3}{5}$$

Drug manufacturers use ratios to express the strengths of injectable drugs, oral solutions and suspensions and topical solutions and topical suspensions.

In compounding, doctors use ratios in prescriptions to express the amount of one ingredient relative to another ingredient. For compounds, doctors often provide the relative ratio of the ingredients and final quantity of the prescription. This is all the information you need to calculate the final quantity of each ingredient in the prescription. The unknown amounts of each ingredient can be determined using a proportion.

Proportions

By setting two ratios equal to each other, you create a proportion.

$$\frac{2}{4} = \frac{4}{8}$$

Considering the left hand side first, 2 divided by 4 equals 0.5. On the right hand side, 4 divided by 8 also equals 0.5, hence these two ratios form a proportion.

As already demonstrated, proportions allow us to calculate an unknown quantity. You will always have three of the four parts of a proportion. By plugging these three known parts into a proportion you can calculate the unknown quantity. The unknown quantity could be the volume of drug that needs to be removed from a stock vial of an injectable drug or the unknown quantity could be an amount of cream or ointment needed to compound a prescription.

Here are the basic steps to using a proportion to calculate an unknown quantity. Let's use the example: a doctor prescribes 200 mg of drug "A" and you have a manufacturer's stock vial that has a concentration of 40 mg/1ml. How many milliliters of drug have 200 mg of drug "A"?

Step1: Setup a proportion with the drug manufacturer's concentration on the left side of the equals sign. Invert the concentration so the "ml" are in the numerator and the "mg" are in the denominator - this will make the math easier.

Step 2: Continuing with setting up the proportion, for the ratio on the right side of the equals sign place an "X" in the numerator to represent the unknown quantity of liquid that has the dose needed. In the denominator, place the dose. Your proportion should like the following:

$$\frac{1 \text{ ml}}{40 \text{ mg}} = \frac{X \text{ ml}}{200 \text{ mg}}$$

Step 3: Cross-multiply both sides by 200 mg. Cross-multiplying erases the 200 mg that is in the denominator on the right side and places it in the numerator on the left side, as follows:

$$\frac{200 \text{ mg} \times 1 \text{ ml}}{40 \text{ mg}} = \frac{X \text{ ml}}{\cancel{200 \text{ mg}}} \times \cancel{200 \text{ mg}}$$

This simplifies to:

$$\frac{200 \text{ mg} \times 1 \text{ ml}}{40 \text{ mg}} = X \text{ ml}$$

The above equation should look familiar to you. It is Method #2 above.

Step 4: Now divide the 200 mg by the 40 mg, which leaves you with:

$$5 \times 1 \text{ ml} = X \text{ ml}$$

Step 5: Simplify this to:

$$5 \text{ ml} = X \text{ ml}$$

Your answer is 5 ml. Many problems can be solved by recognizing that since the 40 mg increased by a factor of 5 to enlarge to 200 mg, then the 1 ml also has to increase by a factor of 5 to 5 ml. This must be true because these are proportions.

Fractions

As you can see by now fractions are very important in pharmaceutical calculations. You need to know how to perform basic mathematical operations with fractions to be able to do pharmaceutical calculations. Therefore, we discuss the basic properties of fractions. 1/2 is a fraction. The "1" is the numerator and the "2" is the denominator. Remember the "d" in denominator stands for "down" or below. You can add, subtract, multiply, and divide fractions.

Adding and Subtracting Fractions

The correct approach to adding or subtracting fractions requires you to have the same denominator in each fraction before adding the numerators. How do you get the denominators to be the same? First, determine if one of the denominators evenly divides into the other denominator without leaving a "remainder." If so, then convert the smaller denominator to the larger denominator and increase the numerator by the same factor. A quick example illustrates this. Add 2/5 and 3/10. First, you have to change the denominator of 5 in 2/5 to a 10 by multiplying by 2. So, you also have to multiply the 2 in the numerator by 2 to keep everything even, which makes it a 4. The 2/5 becomes

4/10, which can be added to the 3/10.

If the smaller denominator doesn't evenly divide into the larger denominator, then proceed to the next step of multiplying the two denominators together. For example, add 2/3 + 1/5. The smaller denominator of 3 does not evenly divide into the larger denominator of 5. You can find a common denominator by multiplying the 3 and 5 together to get 15. Since you multiplied the 3 by 5 to get 15, you also have to multiply the 2 by 5 to get 10, making the new fraction 10/15. Also, since you multiplied the 5 by 3 to get 15, you have to multiply the 1 by 3 to get 3, making the new fraction 3/15. The two fractions are now in the proper form to be added.

Multiplying Fractions

The rules for multiplying fractions are much simpler than the rules for adding and subtracting fractions. You do NOT have to make the denominators the same. For example:

$$\frac{1}{2} \times \frac{1}{2} = \frac{1}{4}$$

The letter "x" represents the multiplication symbol. Although these examples seem trivial, your understanding of the logic behind the answers is crucial.

How about 2/3 x 2/5? Well you simply multiply the numerators together to get 4 and then multiply the denominators together to get 15, so your answer is your new numerator over your new denominator or 4/15. Now can you reduce this fraction of 4/15? No, because there isn't a number that evenly divides both the 4 and the 15 without leaving a remainder.

Dividing Fractions

Dividing fractions is simple. Suppose you want to divide 4/5 by 1/2, what do you do?

$$\frac{4}{5} \div \frac{1}{2} \text{ is the same as } \frac{4}{5} \times \frac{2}{1}$$

Memorize this rule: Dividing by a fraction is the same as multiplying by its "reciprocal." What is a reciprocal? Simply stated, a reciprocal of a fraction is the fraction written upside-down. So if your fraction is 3/5, then its reciprocal is 5/3. If your fraction is 5/7, then its reciprocal is 7/5. Just switch the numerator so it becomes your new denominator and switch your denominator so it becomes your new numerator. That's all there is to it. Now back to our original question: what is 4/5 divided by 1/2. Well you are dividing by 1/2 so the 1/2 is the fraction that you need to switch to its reciprocal. The reciprocal of 1/2 is 2/1 or more simply just 2. So now the problem is 4/5 x 2/1. So now you multiply the 4 and 2 together to get 8 and you multiply the 5 and 1 together to get 5. So now you have 8/5 as your answer.

Use a calculator to check the above answer. First divide 4 by 5 on your calculator. What did you get? 0.8 is the correct answer; so your fraction of 4/5 is equal to 0.8 in decimal format. Now change the 1/2 to decimal format. It is 0.5. On your calculator take 0.8 and divide it by 0.5. What did you get? You got 1.6. Take 8/5 and change it to decimal format. Use your calculator and divide 8 by 5. Did you get 1.6? Well you should have if you typed everything correctly. So you got the same answer of 1.6 each time. These practice questions develop your skills.

Addition

1. $\frac{2}{3} + \frac{3}{7}$

2. $\frac{2}{5} + \frac{2}{8} =$

3. $\frac{3}{8} + \frac{2}{9} =$

4. $\frac{4}{7} + \frac{5}{3} =$

5. $\dfrac{1}{6} + \dfrac{2}{8} =$

6. $\dfrac{1}{3} + \dfrac{2}{4}$

7. $\dfrac{2}{6} + \dfrac{4}{8} =$

8. $\dfrac{2}{9} + \dfrac{2}{4} =$

9. $\dfrac{3}{5} + \dfrac{3}{6} =$

10. $\dfrac{4}{5} + \dfrac{2}{7} =$

11. $\dfrac{3}{7} + \dfrac{2}{9} =$

12. $\dfrac{6}{8} + \dfrac{4}{7} =$

13. $\dfrac{12}{14} + \dfrac{3}{5} =$

14. $\dfrac{11}{7} + \dfrac{1}{2} =$

15. $\dfrac{14}{20} + \dfrac{8}{10} =$

16. $\dfrac{11}{14} + \dfrac{16}{24} =$

17. $\dfrac{16}{14} + \dfrac{5}{3} =$

18. $\dfrac{14}{16} + \dfrac{2}{8} =$

19. $\dfrac{18}{9} + \dfrac{1}{3} =$

20. $\dfrac{15}{20} + \dfrac{1}{5} =$

Subtraction

1. $\dfrac{6}{8} - \dfrac{1}{2} =$

2. $\dfrac{6}{9} - \dfrac{1}{3} =$

3. $\dfrac{3}{4} - \dfrac{1}{2} =$

4. $\dfrac{12}{14} - \dfrac{1}{7} =$

5. $\dfrac{8}{16} - \dfrac{1}{4} =$

6. $\dfrac{4}{10} - \dfrac{1}{5} =$

7. $\dfrac{5}{15} - \dfrac{1}{3} =$

8. $\dfrac{4}{12} - \dfrac{1}{6} =$

9. $\dfrac{3}{9} - \dfrac{1}{3} =$

10. $\dfrac{3}{18} - \dfrac{1}{6}$

Multiplication

1. $\dfrac{1}{2} \times \dfrac{3}{4} =$

2. $\dfrac{1}{2} \times \dfrac{2}{5} =$

3. $\dfrac{1}{3} \times \dfrac{2}{6} =$

4. $\dfrac{1}{4} \times \dfrac{3}{4} =$

5. $\dfrac{2}{3} \times \dfrac{1}{9} =$

6. $\dfrac{2}{4} \times \dfrac{3}{6} =$

7. $\dfrac{3}{5} \times \dfrac{3}{4} =$

8. $\dfrac{4}{5} \times \dfrac{7}{8} =$

9. $\dfrac{4}{6} \times \dfrac{3}{8} =$

10. $\dfrac{3}{7} \times \dfrac{5}{6} =$

11. $\dfrac{4}{9} \times \dfrac{3}{9} =$

12. $\dfrac{3}{12} \times \dfrac{4}{7} =$

13. $\dfrac{2}{18} \times \dfrac{1}{9} =$

14. $\dfrac{4}{16} \times \dfrac{10}{12} =$

15. $\dfrac{3}{15} \times \dfrac{12}{16} =$

16. $\dfrac{8}{24} \times \dfrac{5}{10} =$

17. $\dfrac{12}{16} \times \dfrac{3}{9} =$

18. $\dfrac{15}{20} \times \dfrac{3}{5} =$

19. $\dfrac{16}{18} \times \dfrac{1}{4} =$

20. $\dfrac{12}{4} \times \dfrac{20}{2} =$

Division

1. $\dfrac{2}{3} \div \dfrac{1}{2} =$

2. $\dfrac{4}{8} \div \dfrac{2}{3} =$

3. $\dfrac{1}{7} \div \dfrac{2}{9} =$

4. $\dfrac{2}{8} \div \dfrac{1}{3} =$

5. $\dfrac{2}{6} \div \dfrac{1}{8} =$

6. $\dfrac{4}{5} \div \dfrac{1}{5} =$

7. $\dfrac{6}{8} \div \dfrac{2}{9} =$

8. $\dfrac{4}{8} \div \dfrac{1}{4} =$

9. $\dfrac{2}{5} \div \dfrac{3}{9} =$

10. $\dfrac{6}{9} \div \dfrac{1}{3} =$

11. $\dfrac{10}{12} \div \dfrac{1}{2} =$

12. $\dfrac{12}{14} \div \dfrac{3}{7} =$

13. $\dfrac{12}{16} \div \dfrac{2}{8} =$

14. $\dfrac{12}{18} \div \dfrac{1}{3} =$

15. $\dfrac{14}{42} \div \dfrac{4}{12} =$

16. $\dfrac{18}{27} \div \dfrac{3}{9} =$

17. $\dfrac{16}{32} \div \dfrac{4}{12} =$

18. $\dfrac{16}{8} \div \dfrac{6}{12} =$

19. $\dfrac{12}{4} \div \dfrac{16}{24} =$

20. $\dfrac{24}{3} \div \dfrac{16}{4} =$

Answers

Addition

1. 23/21

2. 13/20

3. 43/72

4. 47/21

5. 5/12

6. 5/6

7. 5/6
8. 13/18

9. 11/10

10. 38/35

11. 41/63

12.   37/28

13.   51/35

14.   29/14

15.   3/2

16.   61/42

17.   59/21

18.   9/8

19.   7/3

20.   19/20

Subtraction

1.   1/4

2.   1/3

3.   1/4

4.   5/7

5.   1/4

6.   1/5

7.   0

8.   1/6

9.   0

10.   0

Multiplication

1.   3/8

2.   1/5

3.   1/9

4.   3/16

5.   2/27

6.   1/4

7.   9/20

8.   7/10

9.   1/4

10.   5/14

11.   4/27

12.   1/7

13.   1/81

14.   5/24

15.   3/20

16.   1/6

17.   1/4

18.	9/20		16.	2
19.	2/9		17.	3/2
20.	30		18.	4

Division

			19.	9/2
1.	4/3		20.	2
2.	3/4			
3.	9/14			
4.	3/4			
5.	8/3			
6.	4			
7.	27/8			
8.	2			
9.	6/5			
10.	2			
11.	5/3			
12.	2			
13.	3			
14.	2			
15.	1			

Chapter 3

Ratio Strengths and Percentage Strengths

What you should learn:

- Understand percentage strength
- Understand ratio strength
- Convert between ratio strength and percentage strength

Percentage Strengths

Generally for injectable drugs and liquid drugs, drug manufacturers label drugs with a concentration of so many milligrams or grams per so many milliliters or liters of liquid. Sometimes however prescription medications may have their strengths listed as percentage strengths or ratio strengths. Specifically how a drug is labeled, percentage strength or ratio strength, tends to be historical and arbitrary, as one can easily convert from one to the other.

Percent refers to the number of parts of something in a total quantity of 100. For example, 5 grams of phenol per every 100 grams of a compound (so that is 5 grams of phenol plus 95 grams of a base). This compound is considered to be 5% because there are 5 grams of drug in 100 grams of the whole compound. Percent is a convenient means of visualizing how much of something exists in every 100 parts of a total substance.

Percentage strengths come in three varieties, percent "volume-in-volume," percent "weight-in-volume," and percent "weight-in-weight." Percent "volume-in-volume" refers to the number of milliliters (ml) of liquid drug in 100 ml of the total solution. It is important to note that the volume of liquid drug is part of the total 100 ml solution; it is not extra. For example, a 100 ml solution that is 5% peppermint oil has 5 ml of peppermint oil and 95 ml of diluent.

Percent "weight-in-volume" refers to the number of grams of drug per 100 ml of total solution. Again, the number of grams of drug is part of the 100 ml of solution. You do not measure out 100 ml of solution and then add 5 grams of drug to it. Rather, you measure out

5 grams of drug, put it in a beaker or graduated cylinder and then add enough water, alcohol, or other liquid to reach the 100 ml mark.

Percent "weight-in-weight" refers to the number of grams of a drug in 100 grams of total compound. For example, 100 grams of a 1% compound of hydrocortisone has 1 gram of hydrocortisone and 99 grams of ointment base. Another example, 50 grams of a 2% compound of phenol in a base has 1 gram of phenol and 49 grams of base.

Ratio Strengths

Ratio strengths may be used when a drug's percentage strength is quite low. Instead of expressing a drug's strength as a percentage strength, you can rewrite it as a ratio strength. For example a drug with a percentage strength of 0.2% can be written as 1:500. Here is the analysis: 0.2% means there are 0.2 grams of drug per 100 grams or 100 ml. For ratio strengths you want to increase that 0.2 grams to the number "1." Here you had to multiply it by 5 to get a "1." Therefore, you multiply the 100 ml by 5 (to maintain the ratio) giving you 500 ml. So your answer is 1:500. Ratio strengths may be used to indicate the strength of medications that are stated as weight-in-volume, volume-in-volume, or weight-in-weight.

Converting From Ratio Strength to Percentage Strength

Practice Problem: Convert 1:3000 to a percentage strength.

Solution: Remember, you want to find the number of parts per 100 parts to find the percentage strength. So you have three of the four parts of a proportion and you just have to solve for the unknown, which is the number of parts in 100 parts.

Initially, 1:3000 equals $\dfrac{1 \text{ part}}{3000 \text{ parts}}$

To determine a percentage, we have to determine how many parts are in 100. So we setup the following proportion to determine the number of parts in 100:

$$\frac{1 \text{ part}}{3000 \text{ parts}} = \frac{X \text{ parts}}{100 \text{ parts}}$$

You can use the same procedure used earlier to calculate drug volumes in Chapter 2 or you can recognize that 3000 parts was divided by 30 to get 100 parts so 1 part has to also be divided by 30, giving you the answer of 0.033%.

Isolate X parts by multiplying both sides by 100 parts, as follows:

$$\frac{100 \text{ parts} \times 1 \text{ part}}{3000 \text{ parts}} = \frac{X \text{ parts}}{100 \text{ parts}} \times 100 \text{ parts}$$

Simplify to:

$$\frac{100 \text{ parts} \times 1 \text{ part}}{3000 \text{ parts}} = X \text{ parts}$$

Simplify by dividing 100 parts by 3000 parts to:

$$0.033 \text{ parts} \times 1 \text{ part} = X \text{ parts}$$

Simplifying again yields:

$$0.033 \text{ parts} = X \text{ parts}$$

So we have 0.033 parts in every 100 parts, which translates to 0.033%. Or, 1:3000 equals 0.033%.

Converting From Percentage Strength to Ratio Strength

Practice Problem: Convert 0.3% to a ratio strength.

0.3% means there are 0.3 parts per 100 parts. As a percentage, we write this as:

$$\frac{0.3\%}{100\%}$$

Remember, with ratio strengths we want to know the amount of solution that contains "1" whole part of drug. With this problem, we know that there are 0.3 parts in 100 ml of solution. We need to convert that 0.3 part into "1" whole part. Well, you have to multiply 0.3 by 3.33 to enlarge it to 1 whole part. Since we multiplied the 0.3 parts by 3.33 to enlarge it, we must also multiply the 100 ml of solution by 3.33 to arrive at the quantity of solution that contains 1 whole part drug. Here that means 333 milliliters contains 1 whole part of drug.

Expressed using a proportion, we have:

$$\frac{0.3\%}{100\%} = \frac{1 \text{ part}}{X \text{ parts}}$$

Multiply both sides by X parts:

$$\frac{X \text{ parts} \times 0.3\%}{100\%} = \frac{1 \text{ part}}{X \text{ parts}} \times X \text{ parts}$$

This simplifies to:

$$\frac{X \text{ parts} \times 0.3\%}{100\%} = 1 \text{ part}$$

Multiply both sides by 100%:

$$100\% \times \frac{X \text{ parts} \times 0.3\%}{100\%} = 1 \text{ part} \times 100\%$$

This simplifies to:

$$X \text{ parts} \times 0.3\% = 1 \text{ part} \times 100\%$$

Now divide both sides by 0.3%:

$$X \text{ parts} \times \frac{0.3\%}{0.3\%} = 1 \text{ part} \times \frac{100\%}{0.3\%}$$

This simplifies to:

$$X \text{ parts} = 1 \text{ part} \times 333$$

Finally,   X parts = 333 parts

Therefore, our answer is 1:333 milliliters.

General Formula for Converting from Percentage Strength to Ratio Strength:

$$X \text{ parts} = 1 \text{ part} \times \frac{100\%}{\text{Percent of solution given in problem}}$$

Review

Drug concentrations can be expressed several ways including the commonly used milligrams per 1 ml, ratio strengths, and percentage strengths. You can convert from one of these to the others with a few simple steps. Ratio strengths are convenient alternatives to percentage strengths. Ratio strengths are used when the percentage strength of a drug is a small decimal number - it is easier to read written as a ratio strength (1:1000) than as a percentage strength. Epinephrine is sometimes expressed as a ratio strength. Lidocaine is commonly expressed as a percentage strength. Percentage strength can be used to describe weight-in weight formulations, weight-in-volume formulations, and volume-in-volume formulations.

Practice Problems:

1)   Change 0.4% into a ratio strength.

2)   Change 0.5% into a ratio strength.

3)   Change 0.65% into a ratio strength.

4)   Change 0.001% into a ratio strength.

5)   Change 0.2% into a ratio strength.

6)   Change 1:1000 into a percentage strength.

7)   Change 1:2000 into a percentage strength.

8)   Change 1:3500 into a percentage strength.

9)   Change 1:10,000 into a percentage strength.

10)   Change 1:200 into a percentage strength.

Answers:

1)   0.4% means there are 0.4 grams in 100 ml of solution. Write a proportion as:

$$\frac{0.4\,\%}{100\,\%} = \frac{1\ \text{part}}{X\ \text{parts}}$$

Isolate X parts by multiplying both sides by X parts, yielding:

$$\frac{X\ \text{parts} \times 0.4\%}{100\%} = \frac{1\ \text{part}}{\cancel{X\ \text{parts}}} \times \cancel{X\ \text{parts}}$$

Simplify this to:

$$\frac{X\ \text{parts} \times 0.4\%}{100\%} = 1\ \text{part}$$

Now multiply both sides by 100% to bring it to the right side, allowing you to start isolating X parts so you can calculate its value:

$$\cancel{100\%} \times \frac{X\ \text{parts} \times 0.4\%}{\cancel{100\%}} = 1\ \text{part} \times 100\%$$

This simplifies to:

$$X\ \text{parts} \times 0.4\% = 1\ \text{part} \times 100\%$$

Finally, isolate X parts by dividing both sides by 0.4%, leaving you with:

$$\text{X parts} \times \frac{\cancel{0.4\%}}{\cancel{0.4\%}} = 1 \text{ part} \times \frac{100\%}{0.4\%}$$

This simplifies to:

$$\text{X parts} = 1 \text{ part} \times 250$$

Finally,
$$\text{X parts} = 250 \text{ parts}$$

Your answer is 1:250. Remember, with ratio strengths, by definition, we want to find how many milliliters have "1" whole part (grams, milligrams, milliliters). You are converting the 0.4 grams to 1 gram and then increasing the volume of 100 ml by the same factor, which is 2.5 in this example.

2) 0.5% means there are 0.5 grams in 100 ml of solution. Write a proportion as:
$$\frac{0.5 \text{ g}}{100 \text{ ml}} = \frac{1 \text{ part}}{\text{X parts}}$$

Isolate X parts by multiplying both sides by X parts, yielding:

$$\frac{\text{X parts} \times 0.5 \text{ g}}{100 \text{ ml}} = \frac{1 \text{ part}}{\cancel{\text{X parts}}} \times \cancel{\text{X parts}}$$

Simplify this to:
$$\frac{\text{X parts} \times 0.5 \text{ g}}{100 \text{ ml}} = 1 \text{ part}$$

Now multiply both sides by 100 ml to bring it to the right side, allowing you to start isolating X parts so you can calculate its value:

Page 46

$$100 \text{ ml} \times \frac{X \text{ parts} \times 0.5 \text{ g}}{100 \text{ ml}} = 1 \text{ part} \times 100 \text{ ml}$$

This simplifies to:

$$X \text{ parts} \times 0.5 \text{ g} = 1 \text{ part} \times 100 \text{ ml}$$

Finally, isolate X parts by dividing both sides by 0.5 grams, leaving you with:

$$X \text{ parts} \times \frac{0.5 \text{ g}}{0.5 \text{ g}} = \frac{1 \text{ part} \times 100 \text{ ml}}{0.5 \text{ g}}$$

This simplifies to:

$$X \text{ parts} = 2 \times 100 \text{ ml}$$

Finally,

$$X \text{ parts} = 200 \text{ ml}$$

Your answer is 1:200. Or, there is one whole part in every 200 ml of solution.

3)   0.65% means there are 0.65 grams in 100 ml of solution. Write a proportion as:

$$\frac{0.65 \text{ g}}{100 \text{ ml}} = \frac{1 \text{ part}}{X \text{ parts}}$$

Isolate X parts by multiplying both sides by X parts, yielding:

$$\frac{X \text{ parts} \times 0.65 \text{ g}}{100 \text{ ml}} = \frac{1 \text{ part}}{X \text{ parts}} \times X \text{ parts}$$

Simplify this to:

$$\frac{X \text{ parts} \times 0.65 \text{ g}}{100 \text{ ml}} = 1 \text{ part}$$

Now multiply both sides by 100 ml to bring it to the right side, allowing you to start isolating X parts so you can calculate its value:

$$\cancel{100\ ml} \times \frac{X\ parts \times 0.65\ g}{\cancel{100\ ml}} = 1\ part \times 100\ ml$$

This simplifies to:

$$X\ parts \times 0.65\ g = 1\ part \times 100\ ml$$

Finally, isolate X parts by dividing both sides by 0.65 grams, leaving you with:

$$X\ parts \times \frac{\cancel{0.65\ g}}{\cancel{0.65\ g}} = \frac{1\ part}{0.65\ g} \times 100\ ml$$

This simplifies to:

$$X\ parts = 1.54 \times 100\ ml$$

Leaving you with:

$$X\ parts = 154\ ml$$

The answer is 1:154. Or, there is one whole part (gram) in every 154 ml of solution. The "part" in "1 part" above can be considered to be "grams" in this context, allowing the "part" and "gram" to cancel each other.

4)   0.001% means there are 0.001 grams in every 100 ml of solution. Write a proportion as:

$$\frac{0.001\ g}{100\ ml} = \frac{1\ part}{X\ parts}$$

Isolate X parts by multiplying both sides by X parts, yielding:

$$\frac{X \text{ parts} \times 0.001 \text{ g}}{100 \text{ ml}} = \frac{1 \text{ part}}{\cancel{X \text{ parts}}} \times \cancel{X \text{ parts}}$$

This simplifies to:

$$\frac{X \text{ parts} \times 0.001 \text{ g}}{100 \text{ ml}} = 1 \text{ part}$$

Multiply both sides by 100 ml so you can further isolate X parts, as follows:

$$\cancel{100 \text{ ml}} \times \frac{X \text{ parts} \times 0.001 \text{ g}}{\cancel{100 \text{ ml}}} = 1 \text{ part} \times 100 \text{ ml}$$

This simplifies to:

$$X \text{ parts} \times 0.001 \text{ g} = 1 \text{ part} \times 100 \text{ ml}$$

Finally, isolate X parts by dividing both sides by 0.001 grams, leaving you with:

$$X \text{ parts} \times \frac{\cancel{0.001 \text{ g}}}{\cancel{0.001 \text{ g}}} = \frac{1 \text{ part}}{0.001 \text{ g}} \times 100 \text{ ml}$$

This simplifies to:

$$X \text{ parts} = 1{,}000 \times 100 \text{ ml}$$

Finally,

$$X \text{ parts} = 100{,}000 \text{ ml}$$

The answer is 1:100,000. Or, there is one whole part (gram) in every 100,000 ml of solution.

5)   0.2% means there are 0.2 grams in every 100 ml of solution. Write a proportion as:

$$\frac{0.2 \text{ g}}{100 \text{ ml}} = \frac{1 \text{ part}}{X \text{ parts}}$$

Isolate X parts by multiplying both sides by X parts, yielding:

$$\frac{X \text{ parts} \times 0.2 \text{ g}}{100 \text{ ml}} = \frac{1 \text{ part}}{\cancel{X \text{ parts}}} \times \cancel{X \text{ parts}}$$

This simplifies to:

$$\frac{X \text{ parts} \times 0.2 \text{ g}}{100 \text{ ml}} = 1 \text{ part}$$

Multiply both sides by 100 ml so you can further isolate X parts, as follows:

$$\cancel{100 \text{ ml}} \times \frac{X \text{ parts} \times 0.2 \text{ g}}{\cancel{100 \text{ ml}}} = 1 \text{ part} \times 100 \text{ ml}$$

This simplifies to:

$$X \text{ parts} \times 0.2 \text{ g} = 1 \text{ part} \times 100 \text{ ml}$$

Finally, isolate X parts by dividing both sides by 0.2 grams, leaving you with:

$$X \text{ parts} \times \frac{\cancel{0.2 \text{ g}}}{\cancel{0.2 \text{ g}}} = \frac{1 \text{ part}}{0.2 \text{ g}} \times 100 \text{ ml}$$

This simplifies to:

$$X \text{ parts} = 5 \times 100 \text{ ml}$$

Finally,
$$X \text{ parts} = 500 \text{ ml}$$

The answer is 1:500. Or, there is 1 gram in every 500 ml of solution.

6)   1:1000 in ratio strength means there is 1 gram of drug in 1000 ml of solution. Write a proportion as follows:

$$\frac{1 \text{ g}}{1000 \text{ ml}} = \frac{X \text{ grams}}{100 \text{ ml}}$$

Recognize that the 1000 ml on the left side of the equals sign has been decreased by a factor of 10 to 100 ml on the right side, so the 1 gram on the left side also has to be reduced by a factor of 10 to 0.1 grams. So you have 0.1 grams in 100 ml, which makes it a 0.1% solution. Or, you can use a more formalistic approach, as follows:

Isolate X grams by multiplying both sides by 100 ml:

$$\frac{100 \text{ ml} \times 1 \text{ g}}{1000 \text{ ml}} = \frac{X \text{ grams}}{\cancel{100 \text{ ml}}} \times \cancel{100 \text{ ml}}$$

Simplify to:

$$\frac{100 \text{ ml} \times 1 \text{ g}}{1000 \text{ ml}} = X \text{ grams}$$

Divide the 100 ml in the numerator by the 1000 ml in the denominator:

$$0.1 \times 1 \text{ g} = X \text{ grams}$$

Finally,

$$0.1 \text{ g} = X \text{ grams}$$

The answer is 0.1 grams in 100 ml, which makes it a 0.1% solution.

7)   1:2000 in ratio strength means there is 1 gram of drug in 2000 ml of solution. Write a proportion as:

$$\frac{1 \text{ g}}{2000 \text{ ml}} = \frac{X \text{ grams}}{100 \text{ ml}}$$

Isolate X grams by multiplying both sides by 100 ml:

$$\frac{100 \text{ ml} \times 1 \text{ g}}{2000 \text{ ml}} = \frac{X \text{ grams}}{\cancel{100 \text{ ml}}} \times \cancel{100 \text{ ml}}$$

This simplifies to:

$$\frac{100 \text{ ml} \times 1 \text{ g}}{2000 \text{ ml}} = X \text{ grams}$$

Divide the 100 ml by the 2000 ml and simplify:

$$0.05 \times 1 \text{ g} = X \text{ grams}$$

This simplifies to:

$$0.05 \text{ g} = X \text{ grams}$$

The answer is 0.05 grams in 100 ml, which makes it a 0.05% solution.

8)   1:3500 means there is one gram of drug in 3500 ml of solution. Write a proportion as follows:

$$\frac{1 \text{ g}}{3500 \text{ ml}} = \frac{X \text{ grams}}{100 \text{ ml}}$$

Isolate X gram by multiplying both sides by 100 ml, as follows:

$$\frac{100 \text{ ml} \times 1 \text{ g}}{3500 \text{ ml}} = \frac{X \text{ grams}}{\cancel{100 \text{ ml}}} \times \cancel{100 \text{ ml}}$$

This simplifies to:

$$\frac{100 \text{ ml} \times 1 \text{ g}}{3500 \text{ ml}} = X \text{ grams}$$

Divide 100 ml by 3500 ml, yielding:

$$0.029 \times 1 \text{ g} = X \text{ grams}$$

This further simplifies to:

$$0.029 \text{ g} = X \text{ grams}$$

The answer is 0.029 grams in 100 ml, which makes it a 0.029% solution.

9)   1:10,000 in ratio strength means there is one gram of drug in 10,000 ml of solution. Write a proportion as follows:

$$\frac{1 \text{ g}}{10,000 \text{ ml}} = \frac{X \text{ grams}}{100 \text{ ml}}$$

Multiply both sides by 100 ml so you can isolate X gram, as follows:

$$\frac{100 \text{ ml} \times 1 \text{ g}}{10,000 \text{ ml}} = \frac{X \text{ grams}}{\cancel{100 \text{ ml}}} \times \cancel{100 \text{ ml}}$$

This simplifies to:

$$\frac{100 \text{ ml} \times 1 \text{ g}}{10,000 \text{ ml}} = X \text{ grams}$$

Divide 100 ml by 10,000 ml:

$$0.01 \times 1 \text{ g} = X \text{ grams}$$

Finally,

$$0.01 \text{ g} = X \text{ grams}$$

The answer is 0.01 grams in 100 ml, which makes it a 0.01% solution.

10)   1:200 means there is one gram in 200 ml of solution. Write a proportion as follows:

$$\frac{1 \text{ g}}{200 \text{ ml}} = \frac{X \text{ grams}}{100 \text{ ml}}$$

As above, you should recognize that the 200 ml was divided by "2" to get 100 ml, and so the 1 g must also be divided by 2, (to keep everything proportional) resulting in 0.5 g per 100 ml, which makes the answer 0.5%. The algebraic steps follow:

Isolate X grams by multiplying both sides by 100 ml:

$$\frac{100 \text{ ml} \times 1 \text{ g}}{200 \text{ ml}} = \frac{X \text{ grams}}{\cancel{100 \text{ ml}}} \times \cancel{100 \text{ ml}}$$

This simplifies to:

$$\frac{100 \text{ ml} \times 1 \text{ g}}{200 \text{ ml}} = X \text{ grams}$$

Divide the 100 ml by 200 ml:

$$0.5 \times 1 \text{ g} = X \text{ grams}$$

Finally,

$$0.5 \text{ g} = X \text{ grams}$$

The answer is 0.5 gram in 100 ml of solution, which makes it a 0.5% solution.

Chapter 4

Intravenous Therapy

What You Should Learn:

- Calculate infusion rates of IV bags
- Calculate drip rates

Introduction to Intravenous Therapy

Some injectable drugs can be administered as a single intravenous bolus dose or IV push over a few minutes provided that the volume is small enough and the drug can safely be administered fairly quickly. The doses of other injectable drugs must be dissolved in an intravenous bag (IV bag) before they can be injected into a patient. These IV bags usually range in volume between 50 ml and 1000 ml.

Calculating the Flow Rate Per Hour

IV pumps are commonly used to administer IV fluids and intravenous drugs to patients. These pumps require you to enter the volume of milliliters per hour (the rate) that is administered to a patient. Therefore, you must know how to calculate how many ml per hour will be administered to a patient. Calculating the number of ml per hour requires dividing the volume of the IV bag by the hours the IV bag is suppose to be administered over (interval). The volume of the IV bag is decided either by a physician, another clinician, or pharmacist depending on the particular circumstances. Some common intervals include 4 hours, 6 hours, 8 hours, and 12 hours.

$$\text{Rate per hour} = \frac{\text{Volume of the IV bag}}{\text{Hours the IV bag is infused over}}$$

Example Practice Problem:

Calculate the number of ml administered per hour of a 1000 ml IV bag that is administered over 12 hours.

$$\frac{1000 \text{ ml}}{12 \text{ hours}} = \frac{X \text{ ml}}{1 \text{ hour}}$$

Dividing 1000 by 12 provides the answer of 83.3 ml per hour.

$$\frac{1000 \text{ ml}}{12 \text{ hours}} = \frac{83.3 \text{ ml}}{1 \text{ hour}}$$

Calculate the number of ml administered per minute from the same IV bag.

$$12 \text{ hours} = 720 \text{ minutes}$$

$$\frac{1000 \text{ ml}}{720 \text{ minutes}} = \frac{1.39 \text{ ml}}{1 \text{ min}}$$

That is 1.39 ml per minute.

Example Practice Problem:

Calculate the number of ml administered per hour of a 500 ml IV bag that is administered over 4 hours.

$$\frac{500 \text{ ml}}{4 \text{ hours}} = \frac{X \text{ ml}}{1 \text{ hour}}$$

$$\frac{500 \text{ ml}}{4 \text{ hours}} = \frac{125 \text{ ml}}{1 \text{ hour}}$$

That is 125 ml per hour.

Calculate the number of ml administered per minute when a

500 ml IV bag is administered over 4 hours.

$$\frac{500 \text{ ml}}{240 \text{ minutes}} = \frac{2.08 \text{ ml}}{1 \text{ minute}}$$

Example Practice Problem:

Calculate the number of ml administered per hour when a 1000 ml IV bag is administered over 4 hours.

$$\frac{1000 \text{ ml}}{4 \text{ hours}} = \frac{X \text{ ml}}{1 \text{ hour}}$$

$$\frac{1000 \text{ ml}}{4 \text{ hours}} = \frac{250 \text{ ml}}{1 \text{ hour}}$$

Calculate the number of ml administered per minute when a 1000 ml IV bag is administered over 4 hours.

$$\frac{1000 \text{ ml}}{240 \text{ minutes}} = \frac{4.17 \text{ ml}}{1 \text{ min}}$$

Calculating the Drip Rate

The drip rate is used to measure the number of ml administered per minute to a patient when an IV pump is not used. An IV pump can accurately measure the number of ml administered per minute or hour. However, an IV pump is not always used, and that means you have to have another way of measuring the number of ml administered per minute or hour.

You measure the number of ml administered per minute by counting the number of drops dropping each minute into a drip chamber (part of the tubing that connects an IV bag to a patient). In general, depending on the specific IV tubing set, 10 drops equals 1 ml, or 15 drops equals 1 ml, or 20 drops equals 1 ml, or 60 drops equals 1 ml.

Instead of thinking of an IV bag as having 1000 ml of solution, think of that same IV bag as having 10,000, or 15,000 or 20,000 or 60,000 drops of solution. In general, each 1 ml of solution is made of about 10, 15, 20, or 60 drops on average, depending on the tubing set used. So by counting the number of drops dropping into a drip chamber each minute, you know the number of ml per minute that is administered to a patient.

There is no practical way to measure 2 ml or 3 ml or 4 ml leaving a 500 ml or 1,000 ml IV bag each minute - a plastic IV bag is not like a glass graduated cylinder - it is simply too difficult to know that 2 ml or 3 ml or 4 ml have left a bag each minute. The number of drops falling by gravity each minute is a practical way of measuring the number of ml administered each minute.

Equation for Calculating the Drip Rate:

$$\text{Drops per minute} = \frac{\text{Volume of IV in milliliters} \times \text{Drops per 1 ml}}{\text{Infusion time in minutes}}$$

Initially, the abbreviation for "drops" is "gtts". You are provided with all of the information you need for this calculation. A doctor tells you both the volume of the infusion and the infusion time. The IV tubing package tells you the number of drops per 1 ml. All you have to do is identify the values and plug them into the equation.

Example Practice Problem:

A doctor writes an order for 1000 ml of normal saline to be infused over 12 hours. You have tubing that is labeled 20 drops per 1 ml. What is the drip rate per minute?

1)   Convert 12 hours to minutes by multiplying by 60 minutes per hour, as follows:

$$12 \text{ hours} \times \frac{60 \text{ minutes}}{1 \text{ hour}} = 720 \text{ minutes}$$

2)   Convert 1000 ml to drops, as follows:

$$1000 \text{ ml} \times \frac{20 \text{ drops}}{1 \text{ ml}} = 20{,}000 \text{ drops}$$

3)   Now, divide 20,000 drops by 720 minutes to determine the number of drops per minute:

$$\frac{20{,}000 \text{ drops}}{720 \text{ minutes}} = \frac{27.8 \text{ drops}}{1 \text{ minute}}$$

You cannot have a fraction of a drop, so round-up to 28 drops per minute.

Example Practice Problem:

A doctor writes an order for 500 ml of D5W (dextrose 5% in water) to be infused over 8 hours. You have tubing that is labeled 10 drops per 1 ml. What is the drip rate per minute?

1)   Convert 8 hours to minutes by multiplying by 60 minutes per hour as follows:

$$8 \text{ hours} \times \frac{60 \text{ minutes}}{1 \text{ hour}} = 480 \text{ minutes}$$

2)   Convert 500 ml to drops:

$$500 \text{ ml} \times \frac{10 \text{ drops}}{1 \text{ ml}} = 5000 \text{ drops}$$

3)   Now divide 5000 drops by 480 minutes to determine the number of drops per minute:

$$\frac{5000 \text{ drops}}{480 \text{ minutes}} = \frac{10.4 \text{ drops}}{1 \text{ minute}}$$

The answer is 10 drops per minute. Here, you round down because the decimal (0.4) is less than 5.

Review
IVs can be administered by an IV pump or by gravity. Use of

an IV pump may require you to calculate the number of ml administered per hour. Calculate the number of ml administered per hour by dividing the volume of the IV by the number of hours the IV is administered over. IVs administered by gravity require you to calculate the drip rate, which is the number of drops dropping per minute. The number of drops dropping per minute equals a certain number of ml per minute. Each IV tubing set is labeled indicating how many drops equals an ml. Usually, 10 drops equals a ml, or 15 drops equals a ml, or 20 drops equals a ml, or 60 drops equals a ml.

Practice Problems

1)   A medication order reads 1000 ml of normal saline (0.9%) to be administered over 6 hours. The IV tubing is marked 10 drops per 1 ml. What is the drip rate?

2)   A medication order reads 1000 ml of normal saline to be administered over 5 hours. The IV tubing is marked 20 drops per 1 ml. What is the drip rate?

3)   A medication order reads 1000 ml of D5W to be administered over 8 hours. The tubing is marked 15 drops per 1 ml. What is the drip rate?

4)   A medication order reads 750 ml of normal saline to be administered over 4 hours. The IV tubing is marked 15 drops per 1 ml. What is the drip rate?

5)   A medication order reads 750 ml of normal saline to be administered over 6 hours. The tubing is marked 60 drops per 1 ml. What is the drip rate?

6)   A medication order reads 1000 ml of lactated ringers to be administered over 12 hours. The tubing is marked 15 drops per 1 ml. What is the drip rate?

7)   A medication order reads 1000 ml of lactated ringers to be

administered over 8 hours. The tubing is marked 10 drops per 1 ml. What is the drip rate?

8)   A medication order reads 500 ml of D5W to be administered over 3 hours. The IV tubing is marked 20 drops per 1 ml. What is the drip rate?

9)   A medication order reads 500 ml of D5W to be administered over 10 hours. The IV tubing is marked 60 drops per 1 ml. What is the drip rate?

10)   A medication order reads 500 ml of D5W to be administered over 8 hours. The IV tubing is marked 60 drops per 1 ml. What is the drip rate?

ANSWERS:

1)   Use the following formula to calculate the number of drops per minute:

$$\text{Drops per minute} = \frac{\text{Volume of IV in milliliters} \times \text{Drops per 1 ml}}{\text{Infusion time in minutes}}$$

First convert 6 hours to 360 minutes. Now plug the values into the equation:

$$\text{Drops per minute} = \frac{1000 \text{ ml} \times 10 \text{ drops per 1 ml}}{360 \text{ minutes}}$$

Notice that in the numerator the ml for the 1000 ml and the ml for the 10 gtts/ml both cancel each other out, leaving you with the only unit left: drops (gtts).

Simplify to:
$$\text{Drops per minute} = \frac{10,000 \text{ drops}}{360 \text{ minutes}}$$

$$\text{Drops per minute} = \frac{27.7 \text{ drops}}{1 \text{ minute}}$$

The answer is 27.7 drops per minute, but you have to round-up to 28 drops.

2) First, 5 hours = 300 minutes. Now use the formula:

$$\text{gtts/min} = \frac{\text{ml} \times \text{drops/ml}}{\text{minute}}$$

$$\text{gtts/min} = \frac{1000 \text{ ml} \times 60 \text{ gtts/ml}}{300 \text{ minutes}}$$

This simplifies to:

$$\text{gtts/min} = \frac{60,000 \text{ gtts}}{300 \text{ minutes}}$$

$$\text{gtts/min} = \frac{200 \text{ gtts}}{1 \text{ minute}}$$

The answer is 200 drops per minute.

3) First, 8 hours = 480 minutes.

$$\text{gtts/min} = \frac{1000 \text{ ml} \times 15 \text{ gtts/ml}}{480 \text{ minutes}}$$

This simplifies to:

$$\text{gtts/min} = \frac{15,000 \text{ gtts}}{480 \text{ minutes}}$$

$$\text{gtts/min} = \frac{31.25 \text{ gtts}}{1 \text{ minute}}$$

The answer is 31 drops per minute. You round down from 31.25 drops.

4) First, 4 hours = 240 min.

$$\text{gtts/min} = \frac{750 \text{ ml} \times 15 \text{ gtts/ml}}{240 \text{ minutes}}$$

This simplifies to:

$$\text{gtts/min} = \frac{11,250 \text{ gtts}}{240 \text{ minutes}}$$

$$\text{gtts/min} = \frac{46.8 \text{ gtts}}{1 \text{ minute}}$$

The answer is 47 drops per minute; you round-up from 46.8.
5) First, 6 hours = 360 minutes. Now use the formula:

$$\text{gtts/min} = \frac{750 \text{ ml} \times 60 \text{ gtts/ml}}{360 \text{ minutes}}$$

This simplifies to:

$$\text{gtts/min} = \frac{45,000 \text{ gtts}}{360 \text{ minutes}}$$

$$\text{gtts/min} = \frac{125 \text{ gtts}}{1 \text{ minute}}$$

The answer is 125 drops per minute.

6) First, 12 hours = 720 minutes. Now use the formula:

$$\text{gtts/min} = \frac{1000 \text{ ml} \times 15 \text{ gtts/ml}}{720 \text{ minutes}}$$

This simplifies to:

$$\text{gtts/min} = \frac{15{,}000 \text{ gtts}}{720 \text{ minutes}}$$

$$\text{gtts/min} = \frac{20.8 \text{ gtts}}{1 \text{ minute}}$$

The answer is 21 drops per minute after rounding.

7)   First, 8 hours = 480 minutes. Now use the formula:

$$\text{gtts/min} = \frac{1000 \text{ ml} \times 10 \text{ gtts/ml}}{480 \text{ minutes}}$$

This simplifies to:

$$\text{gtts/min} = \frac{10{,}000 \text{ gtts}}{480 \text{ minutes}}$$

$$\text{gtts/min} = \frac{20.8 \text{ gtts}}{1 \text{ minute}}$$

The answer is 21 drops per minute, after rounding.

8)   First, 3 hours = 180 minutes. Now use the formula:

$$\text{gtts/min} = \frac{\text{ml} \times \text{drops/ml}}{\text{minute}}$$

$$\text{gtts/min} = \frac{500 \text{ ml} \times 20 \text{ gtts/ml}}{180 \text{ minutes}}$$

This simplifies to:

$$\text{gtts/min} = \frac{10{,}000 \text{ gtts}}{180 \text{ minutes}}$$

$$\text{gtts/min} = \frac{55.5 \text{ gtts}}{1 \text{ minute}}$$

The answer is 56 drops per minute, after rounding.

9)   First, 10 hours = 600 minutes. Now use the formula:

$$\text{gtts/min} = \frac{500 \text{ ml} \times 60 \text{ gtts/ml}}{600 \text{ minutes}}$$

This simplifies to:

$$\text{gtts/min} = \frac{30,000 \text{ gtts}}{600 \text{ minutes}}$$

$$\text{gtts/min} = \frac{50 \text{ gtts}}{1 \text{ minute}}$$

The answer is 50 drops per minute.

10)   First, 8 hours = 480 minutes. Now use the formula:

$$\text{gtts/min} = \frac{\text{ml} \times \text{drops/ml}}{\text{minute}}$$

$$\text{gtts/min} = \frac{500 \text{ ml} \times 60 \text{ gtts/ml}}{480 \text{ minutes}}$$

This simplifies to:

$$\text{gtts/min} = \frac{30,000 \text{ gtts}}{480 \text{ minutes}}$$

$$\text{gtts/min} = \frac{62.5 \text{ gtts}}{1 \text{ minute}}$$

The answer is 63 drops per minute, after rounding.

Chapter 5

Compounding Prescriptions

What You Should Learn:

- Mixing compounds in equal parts
- Mixing compounds in unequal parts

Introduction to Compounding

Although nurses typically do not compound prescriptions, you may decide to work for a practice that specializes in dermatology. Dermatologists commonly write prescriptions for compounded medications. Understanding how to calculate the quantities of ingredients in compounds will help you work in a dermatology office.

A "compound" is a mixture of two different active pharmaceutical ingredients, usually: 1) two different creams 2) two different ointments 3) one cream and one ointment, or 4) two different liquids. In real life, common ratios of ingredients include 1 to 1; 1 to 2; and 1 to 3. For testing purposes, you may see an unusual ratio of two ingredients.

Here we consider the basics of mixing two creams together to form a compound. The math is the same whether two creams are mixed together or a cream and an ointment are mixed together or two ointments are mixed together.

Getting straight to the point, doctors write prescriptions for compounds giving you the relative amounts of the two ingredients and the final quantity of the total prescription. Almost always, you have to calculate the actual quantities of each ingredient. You use a proportion to "scale up" from the relative amounts provided by the doctor to the final prescription quantity prescribed by a doctor - think of making two cakes from a recipe for one, you double all of the ingredients.

Compounds with Equal Parts: 1 to 1

For example, a prescription states "mix cream "A" and cream "B" 1:1 and dispense 10 grams." Read this as saying, "mix 1 gram of cream

"A" with 1 gram of cream "B". It is probably obvious to you that you need 5 grams of each to make 10 grams, but the answer will not always be obvious. You use the relative amounts of 1:1 to write a ratio "for every 1 gram of cream A, we have 2 grams of total compound AND for every 1 gram of cream B, we have 2 grams of total compound." As a ratio or fraction, this can be written as:

$$\frac{1 \text{ gram of cream A}}{1 \text{ gram of cream A} + 1 \text{ gram of cream B}}$$

and,

$$\frac{1 \text{ gram of cream B}}{1 \text{ gram of cream A} + 1 \text{ gram of cream B}}$$

Both of these can be written as:

$$\frac{1 \text{ gram of cream A}}{2 \text{ grams of compound}}$$

and,

$$\frac{1 \text{ gram of cream B}}{2 \text{ grams of compound}}$$

You can use these ratios along with the final prescription quantity of 10 grams to calculate the quantity of cream A and cream B needed to compound the prescription.

$$\frac{1 \text{ gram of cream B}}{2 \text{ grams of compound}} = \frac{X \text{ grams of cream B}}{10 \text{ grams of compound}}$$

Multiply both sides by 10 grams:

$$\frac{10 \text{ grams of comp.} \times 1 \text{ gram of B}}{2 \text{ grams of compond}} = \frac{X \text{ grams of B}}{\cancel{10 \text{ grams of compound}}} \times \cancel{10 \text{ grams of comp.}}$$

This simplifies to:

$$\frac{10 \text{ grams of compound} \times 1 \text{ gram of B}}{2 \text{ grams of compond}} = \text{X grams of B}$$

Now divide "10 grams of compound" by "2 grams of compound":

$$5 \times 1 \text{ gram of B} = \text{X grams of B}$$

Finally,

$$5 \text{ grams of B} = \text{X grams of B}$$

To calculate the quantity of cream A needed, you can simply subtract the 5 grams of cream B from the 10 grams total to arrive at 5 grams of cream A.

Compounds with Unequal Parts: 1 to 2

A doctor writes a prescription for 120 grams of triamcinolone 0.1% and a cream base mixed 1:2. Triamcinolone is often abbreviated "TAC" How many grams of triamcinolone 0.1% are required? How many grams of cream base are required? Follow these steps:

1)   Recognize that the relative amounts of the two ingredients are 1:2.

2)   Write a ratio expressing the amount of one ingredient relative to BOTH ingredients in lowest possible terms. Our general ratio is:

$$\frac{\text{\# of grams of ingredient A}}{\text{\# of grams of ingredient A + \# of grams of ingredient B}}$$

Here that translates to:

$$\frac{1 \text{ gram of TAC } 0.1\%}{1 \text{ gram of TAC } 0.1\% + 2 \text{ grams of cream base}}$$

Written more simply:

$$\frac{1 \text{ gram TAC } 0.1\%}{3 \text{ grams of compound}}$$

3) Create a proportion by setting the above ratio equal to the ratio of X grams of TAC 0.1% per 120 grams of compound.

$$\frac{1 \text{ gram TAC } 0.1\%}{3 \text{ grams of compound}} = \frac{X \text{ grams TAC } 0.1\%}{120 \text{ grams of compound}}$$

4) Now, solve this proportion the same way you solved proportions in the previous chapters. Multiply both sides by 120 grams of compound:

$$\frac{120 \text{ g of comp.} \times 1 \text{ gram TAC } 0.1\%}{3 \text{ grams of compound}} = \frac{X \text{ grams TAC } 0.1\%}{\cancel{120 \text{ grams of compound}}} \times \cancel{120 \text{ g of comp}}$$

This simplifies to:

$$\frac{120 \text{ g of comp.} \times 1 \text{ gram TAC } 0.1\%}{3 \text{ grams of compound}} = X \text{ grams TAC } 0.1\%$$

Divide "120 grams of compound" by "3 grams of compound":

$$40 \times 1 \text{ gram of TAC } 0.1\% = X \text{ grams TAC } 0.1\%$$

Finally, $\quad 40 \text{ grams of TAC } 0.1\% = X \text{ grams TAC } 0.1\%$

To calculate the grams of cream base needed, you can subtract 40 grams of TAC 0.1% cream from the total prescription quantity of 120 grams to get 80 grams. Or, you could write another proportion and solve it.

$$\frac{2 \text{ grams of cream base}}{1 \text{ gram of TAC } 0.1\% + 2 \text{ grams of cream base}} = \frac{X \text{ grams of cream base}}{120 \text{ grams of compound}}$$

The above proportion can be written as:

$$\frac{2 \text{ grams of cream base}}{3 \text{ grams of compound}} = \frac{X \text{ grams of cream base}}{120 \text{ grams of compound}}$$

Multiply both sides by 120 g of compound:

$$\frac{120 \text{ g of comp} \times\ 2 \text{ grams of cream base}}{3 \text{ grams of compound}} = \frac{X \text{ grams of cream base}}{\cancel{120 \text{ grams of compound}}} \times \cancel{120 \text{ g of comp.}}$$

This simplifies to:

$$\frac{120 \text{ g of comp} \times\ 2 \text{ grams of cream base}}{3 \text{ grams of compound}} = X \text{ grams of cream base}$$

Divide "120 g of comp" by "3 grams of compound."

$$40 \times 2 \text{ grams of cream base} = X \text{ grams of cream base}$$

Finally, $\quad 80 \text{ grams of cream base} = X \text{ grams of cream base}$

So overall, you need 40 grams of TAC 0.1% cream and 80 grams of cream base.

In place of writing out all of those proportions, you can also follow the following steps. Recognize that there are "three parts" in this prescription. In this example a "part" has a mass measured in grams (if this was a liquid compound then the parts would be ml or liters). One part is TAC 0.1% and two parts are cream base. Divide 120 grams by 3 parts to determine the quantity of each part, which is 40 grams in this example. Since 1 part is TAC 0.1% and one part has a mass of 40 grams then you need 40 grams of TAC 0.1%. Further, since 2 parts are cream base and one part has a mass of 40 grams then you need 80 grams of cream base.

Compounds with Unequal Parts: 1 to 3

A doctor writes a prescription for 120 grams of triamcinolone 0.1% and cream base mixed 1:3. How many grams of triamcinolone 0.1% are required? How many grams of cream base are required? Follow these steps:

1)   Recognize that the relative amounts of the two ingredients are 1:3.

2)   Write a ratio expressing the amount of one ingredient relative to BOTH ingredients in lowest possible terms. Our general ratio is:

$$\frac{\text{\# of grams of ingredient A}}{\text{\# of grams of ingredient A} + \text{\# of grams of ingredient B}}$$

Here that translates to:

$$\frac{1 \text{ gram of TAC } 0.1\%}{1 \text{ gram of TAC } 0.1\% + 3 \text{ grams of cream base}}$$

Written more simply:

$$\frac{1 \text{ gram of TAC } 0.1\%}{4 \text{ grams of compound}}$$

3)   Create a proportion by setting the above ratio equal to the ratio of X grams of TAC per 120 grams of compound.

$$\frac{1 \text{ gram of TAC } 0.1\%}{4 \text{ grams of compound}} = \frac{\text{X grams of TAC } 0.1\%}{120 \text{ grams of compound}}$$

4)   Now, solve this proportion the same way you solved proportions in the previous chapters. Multiply both sides by 120 grams of compound:

$$\frac{120 \text{ g of comp} \times 1 \text{ g of TAC } 0.1\%}{4 \text{ g of compound}} = \frac{\text{X g of TAC } 0.1\%}{\cancel{120 \text{ g of compound}}} \times \cancel{120 \text{ g of comp}}$$

This simplifies to:

$$\frac{120 \text{ g of comp} \times 1 \text{ g of TAC } 0.1\%}{4 \text{ g of compound}} = X \text{ g of TAC } 0.1\%$$

Divide "120 g of compound" by "4 g of compound":

$$30 \times 1 \text{ g of TAC } 0.1\% = X \text{ g of TAC } 0.1\%$$

Finally,

$$30 \text{ g of TAC } 0.1\% = X \text{ g of TAC } 0.1\%$$

So you need 30 grams of TAC 0.1% to make 120 grams of TAC 0.1% and cream base mixed 1:3. Therefore, you need 90 grams of cream base.

Review

For prescriptions, doctors give the relative amount of one ingredient relative to another ingredient. But they do not always provide the final absolute amount of these individual ingredients. BUT, they provide the final amount of the prescription as a whole, 240 grams of cream A, for example. By knowing these two facts: 1) the ratio of the ingredients and 2) the final amount of the prescription, you can calculate the amounts of each ingredient. How? A proportion provides the amount of each ingredient in the prescription. By knowing three of the four pieces of a proportion, you use mathematics to determine the unknown quantity of ingredients.

The above examples are representative of what you will see in actual practice. For test purposes, test writers could give you "1.5 to 2" or "2 to 3" to check whether you understand how to setup the basic formula to calculate the final quantity of individual ingredients. Simply follow the same formula above.

Chapter 6

Insulin Dosing

What You Should Learn:

- **Understand the different types of insulin**
- **Check the concentration on the label**
- **Is the last character a letter "U" or a zero?**

Introduction to Insulin

Insulin, naturally produced by the pancreas, lowers blood sugar. Some people with diabetes require insulin injections to maintain normal blood sugar levels. Insulin is available in numerous different products, including insulin regular, insulin NPH, insulin aspart, insulin glulisine, insulin lispro, insulin detemir, and insulin glargine. Some combination products include:

- Insulin aspart protamine suspension and insulin aspart
- Insulin lispro protamine and insulin lispro, and
- Insulin NPH suspension and insulin regular

Insulin is labeled in terms of "units" not milligrams or grams. All insulin products, except insulin regular, are available only in one strength: "U-100." This means that there are 100 units of insulin in 1 ml of solution or suspension. Insulin Regular is available in U-100 and U-500. U-500 insulin regular has 500 units of insulin per 1 ml.

CHECK THE CONCENTRATION ON THE LABEL

Insulin Regular is available as U-100 and U-500. The U-500 has 5 times the amount of insulin per unit volume than the U-100. If you give someone the U-500 when he or she is suppose to get the U-100, then you will overdose that person by 5 times. You must read the label carefully.

Is the Last Character a Letter "U" or a ZERO?

Sometimes reading the last character in an insulin dose is difficult to do. Sometimes the last character may look like a zero when it is suppose to be a letter "u," leading to a ten-fold overdose. For example, a doctor may write for:

$$\boxed{\text{insulin regular } 9\text{U}}$$

Is this suppose to be 9 units of insulin regular or 90 (ninety) units of insulin regular? If you guess wrong, you will overdose the patient by ten-fold, potentially leading to a fatal error. Always call the doctor whenever in doubt. Do not assume that doctors always write the "u" for units after a dose. If in the above example, the doctor meant 90 units and left off the "u" - assuming you would know that it is units - you would under dose the patient by assuming it is a "U."

Example Practice Problem:

A doctor prescribes insulin NPH 20 units once daily. How many ml of U-100 insulin NPH are needed to provide 20 units? Write a proportion as:

$$\frac{1 \text{ ml}}{100 \text{ units}} = \frac{X \text{ ml}}{20 \text{ units}}$$

Isolate X ml so you can determine its value. Multiply both sides by 20 units as follows:

$$\frac{20 \text{ units} \times 1 \text{ ml}}{100 \text{ units}} = \frac{X \text{ ml}}{20 \text{ units}} \times 20 \text{ units}$$

Simplify to:

$$\frac{20 \text{ units} \times 1 \text{ ml}}{100 \text{ units}} = X \text{ ml}$$

Divide 20 units by 100 units:

$$0.2 \times 1 \text{ ml} = X \text{ ml}$$

Simplify to:

$$0.2 \text{ ml} = X \text{ ml}$$

The answer is 0.2 ml

Example Practice Problem:

A doctor prescribes insulin Regular 84 units twice daily. How many ml of insulin Regular U-100 are needed per dose? Write a proportion as:

$$\frac{1 \text{ ml}}{100 \text{ units}} = \frac{X \text{ ml}}{84 \text{ units}}$$

Isolate X ml so you can determine its value. Multiply both sides by 84 units, as follows:

$$\frac{84 \text{ units} \times 1 \text{ ml}}{100 \text{ units}} = \frac{X \text{ ml}}{\cancel{84 \text{ units}}} \times \cancel{84 \text{ units}}$$

This simplifies to:

$$\frac{84 \text{ units} \times 1 \text{ ml}}{100 \text{ units}} = X \text{ ml}$$

Divide the 84 units by 100 units, as follows:

$$0.84 \times 1 \text{ ml} = X \text{ ml}$$

Finally,

$$0.84 \text{ ml} = X \text{ ml}$$

The answer is 0.84 ml.

Review

Insulin is used to lower blood sugar. Insulin is available in several different formulations. You need to carefully read insulin labels to ensure that you are giving the correct insulin to a patient. All insulin except insulin regular is only available in U-100, which means there are 100 units of insulin in 1 ml. Insulin regular is available in U-100 and U-500, which has 500 units per 1 ml.

Practice Problems:

1) A doctor prescribes insulin Aspart 5 units before meals. How many ml are needed to administer 5 units?

2) A doctor prescribes insulin Glulisine 17 units before meals. How many ml are needed for this dose?

3) A doctor prescribes insulin Regular 125 units three times daily. How many ml are needed of U-100 for this dose?

4) A doctor prescribes insulin Regular 125 units once daily. How many ml are needed of U-500 for this dose?

5) A doctor prescribes insulin Detemir 47 units once daily. How many ml are needed for this dose?

6) A doctor prescribes insulin Glargine 39 units once daily. How many ml are needed for this dose?

7) A nurse practitioner prescribes insulin Regular 137 units once daily. How many ml of U-500 are needed for this dose?

8) A nurse practitioner prescribes insulin Regular 18 units three times daily. How many ml of U-100 is the patient using total each day?

9) A nurse practitioner prescribes insulin Lispro 41 units three times daily. How many ml is the patient using each day?

10)   A nurse practitioner prescribes insulin Glulisine 52 units three times daily.   How many total units is the patient using each day?

Answers:

1)   Write a proportion as follows:

$$\frac{1 \text{ ml}}{100 \text{ units}} = \frac{X \text{ ml}}{5 \text{ units}}$$

Isolate X ml by multiplying both sides by 5 units as follows:

$$\frac{5 \text{ units} \times 1 \text{ ml}}{100 \text{ units}} = \frac{X \text{ ml}}{5 \text{ units}} \times 5 \text{ units}$$

This simplifies to:

$$\frac{5 \text{ units} \times 1 \text{ ml}}{100 \text{ units}} = X \text{ ml}$$

Divide 5 units by 100 units, yielding:

$$0.05 \times 1 \text{ ml} = X \text{ ml}$$

Finally,

$$0.05 \text{ ml} = X \text{ ml}$$

The answer is 0.05 ml.

2)   Write a proportion as follows:

$$\frac{1 \text{ ml}}{100 \text{ units}} = \frac{X \text{ ml}}{17 \text{ units}}$$

Isolate X ml by multiplying both sides by 17 units:

$$\frac{17 \text{ units} \times 1 \text{ ml}}{100 \text{ units}} = \frac{X \text{ ml}}{17 \text{ units}} \times 17 \text{ units}$$

This simplifies to:

$$\frac{17 \text{ units} \times 1 \text{ ml}}{100 \text{ units}} = X \text{ ml}$$

Divide 17 units by 100 units, yielding:

$$0.17 \times 1 \text{ ml} = X \text{ ml}$$

Finally,

$$0.17 \text{ ml} = X \text{ ml}$$

The answer is 0.17 ml.

3)   Write a proportion as follows:

$$\frac{1 \text{ ml}}{100 \text{ units}} = \frac{X \text{ ml}}{125 \text{ units}}$$

Isolate X ml by multiplying both sides by 125 units, yielding:

$$\frac{125 \text{ units} \times 1 \text{ ml}}{100 \text{ units}} = \frac{X \text{ ml}}{\cancel{125 \text{ units}}} \times \cancel{125 \text{ units}}$$

This simplifies to:

$$\frac{125 \text{ units} \times 1 \text{ ml}}{100 \text{ units}} = X \text{ ml}$$

Divide 125 units by 100 units, resulting in:

$$1.25 \times 1 \text{ ml} = X \text{ ml}$$

Finally,

$$1.25 \text{ ml} = X \text{ ml}$$

The answer is 1.25 ml.

4)   Write a proportion as follows:

$$\frac{1 \text{ ml}}{500 \text{ units}} = \frac{X \text{ ml}}{125 \text{ units}}$$

Multiply both sides by 125 units, so X ml can be isolated, as follows:

$$\frac{125 \text{ units} \times 1 \text{ ml}}{500 \text{ units}} = \frac{X \text{ ml}}{\cancel{125 \text{ units}}} \times \cancel{125 \text{ units}}$$

This simplifies to:

$$\frac{125 \text{ units} \times 1 \text{ ml}}{500 \text{ units}} = X \text{ ml}$$

Divide 125 units by 500 units, resulting in:

$$0.25 \times 1 \text{ ml} = X \text{ ml}$$

Finally, $0.25 \text{ ml} = X \text{ ml}$

The dose is 0.25 ml.

5)   Write a proportion as follows:

$$\frac{1 \text{ ml}}{100 \text{ units}} = \frac{X \text{ ml}}{47 \text{ units}}$$

Multiply both sides by 47 units so you can isolate X ml, as follows:

$$\frac{47 \text{ units} \times 1 \text{ ml}}{100 \text{ units}} = \frac{X \text{ ml}}{\cancel{47 \text{ units}}} \times \cancel{47 \text{ units}}$$

This simplifies to:

$$\frac{47 \text{ units} \times 1 \text{ ml}}{100 \text{ units}} = X \text{ ml}$$

Divide the 47 units by 100 units, yielding:

$$0.47 \times 1 \text{ ml} = X \text{ ml}$$

Finally, $\quad\quad 0.47 \text{ ml} = X \text{ ml}$

The answer is 0.47 ml.

6)   Write a proportion as follows:

$$\frac{1 \text{ ml}}{100 \text{ units}} = \frac{X \text{ ml}}{39 \text{ units}}$$

Multiply both sides by 39 units:

$$\frac{39 \text{ units} \times 1 \text{ ml}}{100 \text{ units}} = \frac{X \text{ ml}}{\cancel{39 \text{ units}}} \times \cancel{39 \text{ units}}$$

This simplifies to:

$$\frac{39 \text{ units} \times 1 \text{ ml}}{100 \text{ units}} = X \text{ ml}$$

Divide 39 units by 100 units, resulting in:

$$0.39 \times 1 \text{ ml} = X \text{ ml}$$

Finally, $\qquad$ 0.39 ml = X ml

The answer is 0.39 ml.

7) Write a proportion as follows:

$$\frac{1 \text{ ml}}{500 \text{ units}} = \frac{X \text{ ml}}{137 \text{ units}}$$

Multiply both sides by 137 units so you can isolate X ml, as follows:

$$\frac{137 \text{ units} \times 1 \text{ ml}}{500 \text{ units}} = \frac{X \text{ ml}}{137 \text{ units}} \times 137 \text{ units}$$

This simplifies to:

$$\frac{137 \text{ units} \times 1 \text{ ml}}{500 \text{ units}} = X \text{ ml}$$

Divide 137 units by 500 units, yielding:

$$0.274 \times 1 \text{ ml} = X \text{ ml}$$

Finally, $\qquad$ 0.274 ml = X ml

The answer is 0.274 ml.

8) Write a proportion as follows:

$$\frac{1 \text{ ml}}{100 \text{ units}} = \frac{X \text{ ml}}{18 \text{ units}}$$

Multiply both sides by 18 units:

$$\frac{18 \text{ units} \times 1 \text{ ml}}{100 \text{ units}} = \frac{X \text{ ml}}{18 \text{ units}} \times = 18 \text{ units}$$

This simplifies to:

$$\frac{18 \text{ units} \times 1 \text{ ml}}{100 \text{ units}} = X \text{ ml}$$

Divide 18 units by 100 units, resulting in:

$$0.18 \times 1 \text{ ml} = X \text{ ml}$$

Finally, $0.18 \text{ ml} = X \text{ ml}$

The patient is using 0.18 ml. for each dose or a total of 0.54 ml total daily.

9)   Write a proportion as follows:

$$\frac{1 \text{ ml}}{100 \text{ units}} = \frac{X \text{ ml}}{41 \text{ units}}$$

Multiply both sides by 41 units, yielding:

$$\frac{41 \text{ units} \times 1 \text{ ml}}{100 \text{ units}} = \frac{X \text{ ml}}{\cancel{41 \text{ units}}} \times \cancel{41 \text{ units}}$$

This simplifies to:

$$\frac{41 \text{ units} \times 1 \text{ ml}}{100 \text{ units}} = X \text{ ml}$$

Divide 41 units by 100 units, resulting in:

$$0.41 \times 1 \text{ ml} = X \text{ ml}$$

Finally,   0.41 ml = X ml

The patient uses 0.41 ml for each dose or 1.23 ml total daily.

10)   Write a proportion as follows:

$$\frac{1 \text{ ml}}{100 \text{ units}} = \frac{X \text{ ml}}{52 \text{ units}}$$

Multiply both sides by 52 units so X ml can be isolated, as follows:

$$\frac{52 \text{ units} \times 1 \text{ ml}}{100 \text{ units}} = \frac{X \text{ ml}}{\cancel{52 \text{ units}}} \times \cancel{52 \text{ units}}$$

This simplifies to:

$$\frac{52 \text{ units} \times 1 \text{ ml}}{100 \text{ units}} = X \text{ ml}$$

Divide 52 units by 100 units, yielding:

$$0.52 \times 1 \text{ ml} = X \text{ ml}$$

Finally,   0.52 ml = X ml

The patient uses 0.52 ml in each dose or 1.56 ml total daily.

Chapter 7

Heparin Dosing

What You Should Learn:

- **Introduction to heparin**
- **Common heparin doses and heparin products**
- **Calculate various quantities related to heparin dosing**

Introduction

Heparin prevents blood-clots from forming. It is used to treat thromboembolic disorders and certain myocardial infarctions. "Antithrombin III" stops certain enzymes from creating blood clots. Heparin increases antithrombin's III ability to prevent blood clots.

Heparin can cause bleeding when overdosed. Because heparin can cause bleeding doctors monitor the "activated partial thromboplastin time (aPTT). The aPTT is one of several measures used to monitor how long it takes blood to clot. When a patient on heparin has a prolonged aPTT (taking too long to clot), protamine is administered. Protamine physically binds to heparin, preventing heparin from working, thus decreasing the amount of time a patient takes to clot.

Heparin, like insulin, is measured in USP units (United States Pharmacopoeia units). Several years ago, there used to be a distinction between USP units and international units used in Europe and elsewhere, this distinction no longer exists. (There are about 150 heparin units per mg.)

Common Heparin Doses

Heparin doses vary depending on the condition being treated. Patients with unstable angina/non-ST-elevation myocardial infarction (NSTEMI) are generally administered a bolus dose of 4000 units or 60 units per kilogram and then are administered a constant infusion of 12 units per kilogram per hour. Patients with venous thromboembolism are generally administered a bolus dose of 5000 units or 80 units per kilogram and then are administered a constant infusion of 18 units per kilogram per hour. You must convert the patient's weight in pounds to kilograms to prevent severely overdosing the patient.

Heparin Products

Heparin vials, syringes, and premixed IV bags are available in a wide assortment of strengths and sizes. You must carefully read each label to ensure you are administering the correct dose to your patient. Heparin is available in premixed IV bags from manufacturers in various strengths. For example, heparin sodium is available in 1/2 normal saline (0.45%) with 25,000 units per 250 ml or 500ml. It is also available in D5W as 10,000 units per 250 ml, 20,000 units per 500 ml, and 25,000 units per 250 ml and 500 ml. Heparin is available in various sizes and strengths in glass vials for use in compounding IV bags. Some sizes and strengths include 1000 units per ml in 1 ml, 10 ml, and 30 ml vials. It is also available in 5000 units per 1 ml and 10 ml; 10,000 units per 1 ml in 1 ml, 4 ml, and 5 ml; and 20,000 units per 1 ml in 1 ml vials. Preservative free heparin is available in 1000 units per ml in 2 ml vials.

Example Practice Problem:

A doctor orders a 5000 unit IV bolus dose of heparin. You have a stock vial of 1000 units per 1 ml. How many ml do you need? Write a proportion as follows:

$$\frac{1 \text{ ml}}{1000 \text{ units}} = \frac{X \text{ ml}}{5000 \text{ units}}$$

Isolate X ml by multiplying both sides by 5000 units, yielding:

$$\frac{5000 \text{ units} \times 1 \text{ ml}}{1000 \text{ units}} = \frac{X \text{ ml}}{\cancel{5000 \text{ units}}} \times \cancel{5000 \text{ units}}$$

This simplifies to:

$$\frac{5000 \text{ units} \times 1 \text{ ml}}{1000 \text{ units}} = X \text{ ml}$$

Divide 5000 units by 1000 units, resulting in:

$$5 \times 1 \text{ ml} = X \text{ ml}$$

Finally,

$$5 \text{ ml} = X \text{ ml}$$

The answer is 5 ml.

Example Practice Problem:

A doctor orders a continuous infusion of 12 units per kilogram per hour for a patient weighing 200 pounds. How many heparin units does the patient need per hour?

First, convert 200 pounds to kilograms, as follows:

$$\frac{1 \text{ kg}}{2.2 \text{ pounds}} = \frac{X \text{ kg}}{200 \text{ pounds}}$$

Isolate X kg by multiplying both sides by 200 pounds, as follows:

$$\frac{200 \text{ pounds} \times 1 \text{ kg}}{2.2 \text{ pounds}} = \frac{X \text{ kg}}{200 \text{ pounds}} \times 200 \text{ pounds}$$

This simplifies to:

$$\frac{200 \text{ pounds} \times 1 \text{ kg}}{2.2 \text{ pounds}} = X \text{ kg}$$

Divide 200 pounds by 2.2 pounds, resulting in:

$$90.9 \times 1 \text{ kg} = X \text{ kg}$$

Finally,

$$90.9 \text{ kg} = X \text{ kg}$$

Now, the doctor ordered 12 units per kilogram, write a proportion as follows:

$$\frac{12 \text{ units}}{1 \text{ kg}} = \frac{X \text{ units}}{90.9 \text{ kg}}$$

Isolate X units by multiplying both sides by 90.9 kg, yielding:

$$\frac{90.9 \text{ kg} \times 12 \text{ units}}{1 \text{ kg}} = \frac{X \text{ units}}{90.9 \text{ kg}} \times 90.9 \text{ kg}$$

This simplifies to:

$$\frac{90.9 \text{ kg} \times 12 \text{ units}}{1 \text{ kg}} = X \text{ units}$$

Divide 90.9 kg by 1 kg, as follows:

$$90.9 \times 12 \text{ units} = X \text{ units}$$

Finally,

$$1090.9 \text{ units} = X \text{ units}$$

The answer is the patient receives 1090.8 units per hour.

Review

Heparin reduces the formation of blood clots by increasing the efficiency of antithrombin III. Heparin, being used for several different medical conditions, has various dosing regimens. For unstable angina/non-ST-elevation myocardial infarction, patients typically receive a bolus dose of 4000 units or 60 units per kilogram and then are administered a constant infusion of 12 units per kilogram per hour. For venous thromboembolism, patients usually receive a bolus dose of 5000 units or 80 units per kilogram and then are administered a constant infusion of 18 units per kilogram per hour. It is important to remember to convert a patient's weight in pounds to kilograms. Otherwise, you will severely overdose the patient.

Practice Problems:

1)   A doctor orders 1090 units per hour of heparin. You have a premixed IV bag of 25,000 units in 250 ml. How many ml per hour does the patient need?

2)   A doctor orders 1000 units per hour of heparin. You have a premixed IV bag of 25,000 units in 500 ml. How many ml per hour does the patient need?

3)   A doctor orders an IV bolus dose of 80 units per kilogram for a patient weighing 100 kilograms. How many units does the patient need?

4)   A doctor orders an IV bolus dose of 80 units per kilogram for a patient weighing 100 kilograms. You have a stock vial of 5000 units per 1 ml. How many ml are required for the dose?

5)   A nurse practitioner orders a constant infusion of 18 units per kilogram per hour for a patient weighing 220 pounds. You have an IV bag from the pharmacy that is labeled 100 units per 1 ml. How many ml per hour should the patient receive?

6)   A nurse practitioner orders a constant infusion of 12 units per

kilogram per hour for a patient weighing 80 kg. You have a premixed IV bag that has 50 units per 1 ml. How many ml per hour should the patient receive?

7)   A doctor orders an IV bolus dose of 60 units per kilogram for a patient weighing 90 kilograms. How many units should the patient receive?

8)   A doctor orders an IV bolus dose of 60 units per kilogram for a patient weighing 90 kilograms. You have a stock vial of 1000 units per 1 ml. How many ml should the patient receive?

9)   A doctor orders an IV bolus dose of 5000 units. You have a stock vial of 1000 units per 1 ml. How many ml should the patient receive?

10)   A patient has been receiving 20 ml of heparin per hour from a premixed IV bag that has 25,000 units in 500 ml. How many units per hour has the patient been receiving?

Answers:

1)   First, convert 25,000 units per 250 ml to units per 1 ml. Write a proportion as follows:

$$\frac{25,000 \text{ units}}{250 \text{ ml}} = \frac{X \text{ units}}{1 \text{ ml}}$$

You can simply reduce the fraction on the left by dividing the numerator and denominator by 250, leaving you with:

$$\frac{100 \text{ units}}{1 \text{ ml}} = \frac{X \text{ units}}{1 \text{ ml}}$$

Or, there are 100 units per 1ml in the premixed IV bag. The dose is

1090 units per hour. Write a proportion to calculate the number of ml needed:

$$\frac{1 \text{ ml}}{100 \text{ units}} = \frac{X \text{ ml}}{1090 \text{ units}}$$

Multiply both sides by 1090 units:

$$\frac{1090 \text{ units} \times 1 \text{ ml}}{100 \text{ units}} = \frac{X \text{ ml}}{\cancel{1090 \text{ units}}} \times \cancel{1090 \text{ units}}$$

This simplifies to:

$$\frac{1090 \text{ units} \times 1 \text{ ml}}{100 \text{ units}} = X \text{ ml}$$

Divide 1090 units by 100 units:

$$10.9 \times 1 \text{ ml} = X \text{ ml}$$

Finally, $10.9 \text{ ml} = X \text{ ml}$

The answer is 10.9 ml.

2)   First, convert 25,000 units per 500 ml to units per 1 ml. Write a proportion as follows:

$$\frac{25,000 \text{ units}}{500 \text{ ml}} = \frac{X \text{ units}}{1 \text{ ml}}$$

You can reduce the fraction on the left by dividing the numerator and denominator both by 500, leaving you with:

$$\frac{50 \text{ units}}{1 \text{ ml}} = \frac{X \text{ units}}{1 \text{ ml}}$$

There are 50 units per 1 ml. The dose is 1000 units per hour. Write a proportion to calculate the number of ml needed per hour:

$$\frac{1 \text{ ml}}{50 \text{ units}} = \frac{X \text{ ml}}{1000 \text{ units}}$$

Here you should recognize that the 50 units in the denominator was multiplied by 20 to get 1000 units in the denominator on the right side, so you must also multiply the 1 ml by 20, leaving you with the answer of 20 ml. Otherwise, you can perform the following steps:

Multiply both sides by 1000 units so X ml can be isolated, as follows:

$$\frac{1000 \text{ units} \times 1 \text{ ml}}{50 \text{ units}} = \frac{X \text{ ml}}{\cancel{1000 \text{ units}}} \times \cancel{1000 \text{ units}}$$

This simplifies to:

$$\frac{1000 \text{ units} \times 1 \text{ ml}}{50 \text{ units}} = X \text{ ml}$$

Divide the 1000 units by the 50 units, leaving you with:

$$20 \times 1 \text{ ml} = X \text{ ml}$$

Finally, $\qquad 20 \text{ ml} = X \text{ ml}$

The answer is 20 ml per hour.

3)   The bolus dose is 80 units/kg and the patient weights 100 kilograms. Write a proportion as follows:

$$\frac{80 \text{ units}}{1 \text{ kg}} = \frac{X \text{ units}}{100 \text{ kg}}$$

Multiply both sides by 100 kg so X units can be isolated, as follows:

$$\frac{100 \text{ kg} \times 80 \text{ units}}{1 \text{ kg}} = \frac{X \text{ units}}{100 \text{ kg}} \times 100 \text{ kg}$$

This simplifies to:

$$\frac{100 \text{ kg} \times 80 \text{ units}}{1 \text{ kg}} = X \text{ units}$$

For completeness, divide the 100 kg by 1 kg so you can remove the units:

$$100 \times 80 \text{ units} = X \text{ units}$$

Finally, $8000 \text{ units} = X \text{ units}$

The patient needs 8,000 units. The ml will depend on the vial used.

4)   Based on the previous question, you know the patient needs 8,000 units. Your vial has 5000 units per 1 ml, so write a proportion, as follows:

$$\frac{1 \text{ ml}}{5000 \text{ units}} = \frac{X \text{ ml}}{8000 \text{ units}}$$

Isolate X ml by multiplying both sides by 8000 units:

$$\frac{8000 \text{ units} \times 1 \text{ ml}}{5000 \text{ units}} = \frac{X \text{ ml}}{\cancel{8000 \text{ units}}} \times \cancel{8000 \text{ units}}$$

This simplifies to:

$$\frac{8000 \text{ units} \times 1 \text{ ml}}{5000 \text{ units}} = X \text{ ml}$$

Divide 8000 units by 5000 units, yielding:

$$1.6 \times 1 \text{ ml} = X \text{ ml}$$

Finally, $1.6 \text{ ml} = X \text{ ml}$

The answer is 1.6 ml.

5) First, convert 220 pounds to kilograms. 1 kilogram = 2.2 pounds. Write a proportion as follows:

$$\frac{1 \text{ kg}}{2.2 \text{ pounds}} = \frac{X \text{ kg}}{220 \text{ pounds}}$$

Multiply both sides by 220 pounds so X kg can be determined:

$$\frac{220 \text{ pounds} \times 1 \text{ kg}}{2.2 \text{ pounds}} = \frac{X \text{ kg}}{\cancel{220 \text{ pounds}}} \times \cancel{220 \text{ pounds}}$$

This simplifies to:

$$\frac{220 \text{ pounds} \times 1 \text{ kg}}{2.2 \text{ pounds}} = X \text{ kg}$$

Divide 220 pounds by 2.2 pounds, yielding:

$$100 \times 1 \text{ kg} = X \text{ kg}$$

Finally, $\qquad 100 \text{ kg} = X \text{ kg}$

The patient weighs 100 kg. Second, determine the number of units per hour the patients needs. The patient weighs 100 kg and is getting 18 units per kg per hour. Write a proportion as:

$$\frac{18 \text{ units}}{1 \text{ kg}} = \frac{X \text{ units}}{100 \text{ kg}}$$

Isolate X units by multiplying both sides by 100 kg, resulting in:

$$\frac{100 \text{ kg} \times 18 \text{ units}}{1 \text{ kg}} = \frac{X \text{ units}}{100 \text{ kg}} \times 100 \text{ kg}$$

Divide the 100 kg by 1 kg so you can cancel the units:

$$100 \times 18 \text{ units} = X \text{ units}$$

Finally, $\qquad 1800 \text{ units} = X \text{ units}$

So the patient needs 1800 units per hour. Third, the IV bag is labeled 100 units per 1 ml. Write a proportion as:

$$\frac{1 \text{ ml}}{100 \text{ units}} = \frac{X \text{ ml}}{1800 \text{ units}}$$

Isolate X ml by multiplying both sides by 1800 units, yielding:

$$\frac{1800 \text{ units} \times 1 \text{ ml}}{100 \text{ units}} = \frac{X \text{ ml}}{\cancel{1800 \text{ units}}} \times \cancel{1800 \text{ units}}$$

This simplifies to:

$$\frac{1800 \text{ units} \times 1 \text{ ml}}{100 \text{ units}} = X \text{ ml}$$

Divide 1800 units by 100 units:

$$18 \times 1 \text{ ml} = X \text{ ml}$$

Finally, $18 \text{ ml} = X \text{ ml}$

The patient needs 18 ml per hour.

6)   The patient weighs 80 kg and is receiving 12 units/kg per hour. Write a proportion to determine the number of units infused per hour.

$$\frac{12 \text{ units}}{1 \text{ kg}} = \frac{X \text{ units}}{80 \text{ kg}}$$

Multiply both sides by 80 kg:

$$\frac{80 \text{ kg} \times 12 \text{ units}}{1 \text{ kg}} = \frac{X \text{ units}}{\cancel{80 \text{ kg}}} \times \cancel{80 \text{ kg}}$$

This simplifies to:

$$\frac{80 \text{ kg} \times 12 \text{ units}}{1 \text{ kg}} = \text{X units}$$

Divide 80 kg by 1 kg so you can remove the units:

$$80 \times 12 \text{ units} = \text{X units}$$

Finally, $960 \text{ units} = \text{X units}$

The patient needs 960 units per hour and each ml in the IV bag has 50 units. Write a proportion as follows to determine the volume needed each hour:

$$\frac{1 \text{ ml}}{50 \text{ unit}} = \frac{\text{X ml}}{960 \text{ units}}$$

Multiply both sides by 960 units:

$$\frac{960 \text{ units} \times 1 \text{ ml}}{50 \text{ unit}} = \frac{\text{X ml}}{\cancel{960 \text{ units}}} \times \cancel{960 \text{ units}}$$

This simplifies to:

$$\frac{960 \text{ units} \times 1 \text{ ml}}{50 \text{ unit}} = \text{X ml}$$

Divide the 960 units by 50 units to yield:

$$19.2 \times 1 \text{ ml} = \text{X ml}$$

Finally, $\qquad$ 19.2 ml = X ml

The patient needs 19.2 ml per hour.

7)   The dose is 60 units per kg and the patient weighs 90 kg, what is the dose? Write a proportion as:

$$\frac{60 \text{ units}}{1 \text{ kg}} = \frac{X \text{ units}}{90 \text{ kg}}$$

Multiply both sides by 90 kg:

$$\frac{90 \text{ kg} \times 60 \text{ units}}{1 \text{ kg}} = \frac{X \text{ units}}{90 \text{ kg}} \times 90 \text{ kg}$$

This simplifies to:

$$\frac{90 \text{ kg} \times 60 \text{ units}}{1 \text{ kg}} = X \text{ units}$$

Divide 90 kg by 1 kg so you can remove the units:

$$90 \times 60 \text{ units} = X \text{ units}$$

Finally, $\qquad$ 5400 units = X units

The patient needs 5400 units.

8)   We know from the previous question that the dose is 5400 units. The stock vial has 1000 units per 1 ml. Calculate the number of ml to administer as follows:

$$\frac{1 \text{ ml}}{1000 \text{ units}} = \frac{X \text{ ml}}{5400 \text{ units}}$$

Multiply both sides by 5400 units:

$$\frac{5400 \text{ units} \times 1 \text{ ml}}{1000 \text{ units}} = \frac{X \text{ ml}}{\cancel{5400 \text{ units}}} \times \cancel{5400 \text{ units}}$$

This simplifies to:

$$\frac{5400 \text{ units} \times 1 \text{ ml}}{1000 \text{ units}} = X \text{ ml}$$

Divide 5400 units by 1000 units:

$$5.4 \times 1 \text{ ml} = X \text{ ml}$$

Finally, $5.4 \text{ ml} = X \text{ ml}$

The patient needs 5.4 ml.

9)   The IV bolus dose is 5000 units and the stock vial is 1000 units per 1 ml. Write a proportion as:

$$\frac{1 \text{ ml}}{1000 \text{ units}} = \frac{X \text{ ml}}{5000 \text{ units}}$$

Multiply both sides by 5000 units:

$$\frac{5000 \text{ units} \times 1 \text{ ml}}{1000 \text{ units}} = \frac{X \text{ ml}}{\cancel{5000 \text{ units}}} \times \cancel{5000 \text{ units}}$$

This simplifies to:

$$\frac{5000 \text{ units} \times 1 \text{ ml}}{1000 \text{ units}} = X \text{ ml}$$

Divide 5000 units by 1000 units:

$$5 \times 1 \text{ ml} = X \text{ ml}$$

Finally, $5 \text{ ml} = X \text{ ml}$

The dose is 5 ml.

10)   The IV bag has 25,000 units in 500 ml. First convert that to units per 1 ml as follows:

$$\frac{25{,}000 \text{ units}}{500 \text{ ml}} = \frac{X \text{ units}}{1 \text{ ml}}$$

Reduce the fraction on the left by dividing both the numerator and denominator by 500, resulting in:

$$\frac{50 \text{ units}}{1 \text{ ml}} = \frac{X \text{ units}}{1 \text{ ml}}$$

So there are 50 units per 1 ml in the IV bag. The patient has been receiving 20 ml per hour. How many units are in the 20 ml that the patient receives each hour? Write a proportion as follows:

$$\frac{50 \text{ units}}{1 \text{ ml}} = \frac{X \text{ units}}{20 \text{ ml}}$$

Since the 1ml was multiplied by 20 to get 20 ml, the 50 units must also be multiplied by 20 to keep everything proportional, so the answer is

1000 units. Or, you can write everything out:

Multiply both sides by 20 ml:

$$\frac{20 \text{ ml} \times 50 \text{ units}}{1 \text{ ml}} = \frac{X \text{ units}}{\cancel{20 \text{ ml}}} \times \cancel{20 \text{ ml}}$$

This simplifies to:

$$\frac{20 \text{ ml} \times 50 \text{ units}}{1 \text{ ml}} = X \text{ units}$$

Divide the 20 ml by 1 ml so you can remove the units:

$$20 \times 50 \text{ units} = X \text{ units}$$

Finally, $$1000 \text{ units} = X \text{ units}$$

Again, the answer is 1000 units per hour.

Chapter 8

Calculations Using Body Surface Area

WHAT YOU SHOULD LEARN:

- **Why use Body Surface Area instead of body weight**
- **How to calculate doses based on body surface area**

Introduction to Body Surface Area

Most drugs are usually dosed based on body weight. Body weight is an accurate predictor of the dose a person needs. In some circumstances, doses are based on body surface area (BSA). BSA is considered a better predictor than body weight of the dose a person needs. For children, BSA is commonly used. Many oncology drugs are dosed based on BSA for children and adults alike.

Various complex mathematical formulas exist for calculating BSA for children and adults. Before the widespread use of computers, rather than force clinicians to use time consuming mathematical formulas, nomograms were developed to calculate BSA. Nomograms are charts that allow you to easily determine someone's BSA based on their height and weight. Nomograms consist of three columns. To calculate BSA, you connect a line from the patient's height-marking to the patient's weight-marking, wherever that line crosses the BSA column is the value for the BSA. This book does not endorse any particular nomogram over another and so does not provide specifics about individual nomograms.

Equation for a Kid's Dose based on Body Surface Area

The average adult has a BSA of 1.73 m². Kids' BSAs vary from about 0.1 to sometimes larger than 1.73 m². In general, a kid's BSA is a fraction of the average adult BSA. Therefore, a kid's dose will be that same fraction of the adult dose. However, because of modern diets, some kids have a BSA larger than an average adult's, and, therefore, these kids may have higher doses than adults.

$$\text{Kid's dose} = \frac{\text{Kid's BSA in m}^2}{1.73 \text{ m}^2} \times \text{Adult Dose}$$

Example Practice Problem:

A kid has a BSA of 0.865 m². The adult dose of a drug is 100 mg once daily. What is the kid's dose? Plug the values into the formula, as follows:

$$\text{Kid's dose} = \frac{\text{Kid's BSA in m}^2}{1.73 \text{ m}^2} \times \text{Adult Dose}$$

$$\text{Kid's dose} = \frac{0.865 \text{ m}^2}{1.73 \text{ m}^2} \times 100 \text{ mg}$$

Divide 0.865 m² by 1.73 m², as follows:

$$\text{Kid's dose} = 0.5 \times 100 \text{ mg}$$

Multiply the numbers:

$$\text{Kid's dose} = 50 \text{ mg}$$

Example Practice Problem:

A kid has a BSA of 1.903 m². An adult dose of a drug is 100 mg. What is the kid's dose?

$$\text{Kid's dose} = \frac{\text{Kid's BSA in m}^2}{1.73\text{m}^2} \times \text{Adult Dose}$$

Plug the values into the formula:

$$\text{Kid's dose} = \frac{1.903 \text{ m}^2}{1.73 \text{ m}^2} \times 100 \text{ mg}$$

Divide 1.903 m² by 1.73 m²:

$$\text{Kid's dose} = 1.1 \times 100 \text{ mg}$$

Multiply the numbers:

$$\text{Kid's dose} = 110 \text{ mg}$$

Practice Problems:

1)   A child has a BSA of 1.557 m². The adult dose of a drug is 250 mg. What is the child's dose based on BSA?

2)   A child has a BSA of 1.384 m². The adult dose of a drug is 150 mg. What is the child's dose based on BSA?

3)   A child has a BSA of 1.211 m². The adult dose of a drug is 300 mg. What is the child's dose based on BSA?

4)   A child has a BSA of 1.038 m². The adult dose of a drug is 75 mg. What is the child's dose based on BSA?

5)   A child has a BSA of 0.865 m². The adult dose of a drug is 150

mg. What is the child's dose based on BSA?

6)   A child has a BSA of 0.779 m². The adult dose of a drug is 175 mg. What is the child's dose based on BSA?

7)   A child has a BSA of 1.903 m². The adult dose of a drug is 45 mg. What is the child's dose based on BSA?

8)   A child has a BSA of 1.989 m². The adult dose of a drug is 100 mg. What is the child's dose based on BSA?

9)   A child has a BSA of 2.076 m². The adult dose of a drug is 75 mg. What is the child's dose based on BSA?

10)   A child has a BSA of 2.163 m². The adult dose of a drug is 200 mg. What is the child's dose based on BSA?

Answers:

For all of the questions use the formula:

$$\text{Kid's dose} = \frac{\text{Kid's BSA in m}^2}{1.73\text{m}^2} \times \text{Adult Dose}$$

1)   Write the formula as:

$$\text{Kid's dose} = \frac{1.557 \text{ m}^2}{1.73 \text{ m}^2} \times 250 \text{ mg}$$

$$\text{Kid's dose} = 0.9 \times 250 \text{ mg}$$

$$\text{Kid's dose} = 225 \text{ mg}$$

2)   Write the formula as:

$$\text{Kid's dose} = \frac{1.384 \text{ m}^2}{1.73 \text{ m}^2} \times 150 \text{ mg}$$

Kid's dose = 0.8 × 150 mg

Kid's dose = 120 mg

3)   Write the formula as:

$$\text{Kid's dose} = \frac{1.211 \text{ m}^2}{1.73 \text{ m}^2} \times 300 \text{ mg}$$

Kid's dose = 0.7 × 300 mg

Kid's dose = 210 mg

4)   Write the formula as:

$$\text{Kid's dose} = \frac{1.038 \text{ m}^2}{1.73 \text{ m}^2} \times 75 \text{ mg}$$

Kid's dose = 0.6 × 75 mg

Kid's dose = 45 mg

5)   Write the formula as:

$$\text{Kid's dose} = \frac{0.865 \text{ m}^2}{1.73 \text{ m}^2} \times 150 \text{ mg}$$

$$\text{Kid's dose} = 0.5 \times 150 \text{ mg}$$

$$\text{Kid's dose} = 75 \text{ mg}$$

6)   Write the formula as:

$$\text{Kid's dose} = \frac{0.779 \text{ m}^2}{1.73 \text{ m}^2} \times 175 \text{ mg}$$

$$\text{Kid's dose} = 0.45 \times 175 \text{ mg}$$

$$\text{Kid's dose} = 78.75 \text{ mg}$$

7)   Write the formula as follows:

$$\text{Kid's dose} = \frac{1.903 \text{ m}^2}{1.73 \text{ m}^2} \times 45 \text{ mg}$$

$$\text{Kid's dose} = 1.1 \times 45 \text{ mg}$$

$$\text{Kid's dose} = 49.5 \text{ mg}$$

8)   Write the formula as:

$$\text{Kid's dose} = \frac{1.989 \text{ m}^2}{1.73 \text{ m}^2} \times 100 \text{ mg}$$

Kid's dose = 1.15 $\times$ 100 mg

Kid's dose = 115 mg

9)   Write the formula as:

$$\text{Kid's dose} = \frac{2.076 \text{ m}^2}{1.73 \text{ m}^2} \times 75 \text{ mg}$$

Kid's dose = 1.2 $\times$ 75 mg

Kid's dose = 90 mg

10)   Write the formula as:

$$\text{Kid's dose} = \frac{2.163 \text{ m}^2}{1.73 \text{ m}^2} \times 200 \text{ mg}$$

Kid's dose = 1.25 $\times$ 200 mg

Kid's dose = 250 mg

Chapter 9

Enteral Nutrition and Parenteral Nutrition

WHAT YOU SHOULD LEARN:

- **Enteral nutrition and parenteral nutrition**
- **Parenteral nutrition calculations**

Introduction

Enteral nutrition involves feeding patients through feeding tubes. Enteral nutrition is used when patients have difficulty swallowing. Parenteral nutrition involves the infusion of intravenous solutions of nutrients into a vein. Parenteral nutrition is a last option. Enteral nutrition is preferred over parenteral nutrition because it is generally safer for patients, but sometimes enteral feeding is not possible and parenteral nutrition must be used.

Enteral nutrition products are available by several different manufacturers, who produce many different enteral nutrition products. Considerable variety exists between enteral nutrition products. Products that have a high osmolality may require dilution with water before being used because they can be stressful to a patient's gastrointestinal tract. Diluting products with water increases the risk of introducing harmful bacteria into a patient. So new products were developed that do not require dilution. Diluting enteral nutrition products has become much less common than it used to be. In brief, to dilute enteral nutrition products you:

1) Divide the package size by the percentage strength the physician wants the product administered at. So if the package size is 240 ml and the doctor wants it diluted by 50%, then divide 240 by 0.5 giving you 480 ml.

2) 480 ml is now the new total volume. Subtract the original package size of 240 ml from 480 ml to determine the amount of water that has to be added, in this case 240 ml.

"Total parenteral nutrition," (TPN) is a mixture of nutrients including amino acids (for protein synthesis), lipids, dextrose, vitamins, trace elements, heparin, insulin, and sometimes a histamine H_2 receptor blocker to treat ulcers. The specific ingredients of TPNs vary from patient to patient. Patients with different types of illnesses require different amounts of fluid, carbohydrates, amino acids, and lipids. Heparin is used because the various types of tubing used to infuse TPNs tend to cause blood clots.

The calculations necessary to make an IV bag of a TPN are the same as the calculations that you have already studied. TPNs can have many different ingredients - you separately calculate the volume of each ingredient needed. After calculating the volume of each ingredient, you generally enter those values into a compounding machine that makes the TPN for you. Most pharmacies use compounding machines to produce TPNs. Making a TPN by hand is physically difficult and time consuming.

Daily, the body needs a certain amount of fluids, carbohydrates, amino acids, vitamins, and minerals each day to maintain health. Healthy people generally need about 30 ml of fluid for each one kilogram of body mass. So a 70 kg person needs about 2100 ml of fluid daily to maintain health. Patients with renal problems or cardiac problems may require less fluid per day.

Daily, most healthy people use about 30 kilo-calories of energy per kilogram of body weight. So a 70 kilogram person needs about 2100 kilo-calories daily. Some health conditions can increase a person's daily energy requirements above 30 kilo-calories per kilogram of body weight. Lipids should not account for more than 30% of a person's energy requirements.

TPNs provide energy through amino acids, dextrose, and lipids. Amino acids in general have 4 kilo-calories of energy per gram. Dextrose provides 3.4 kilo-calories per gram. Lipids provide 9 kilo-calories per gram. The amount of amino acids, dextrose, and lipids varies from TPN to TPN. Because the amount of amino acids varies from TPN to TPN, the amount of total energy available from amino acids varies from TPN to TPN and the same holds true for dextrose and lipids.

Patients receiving TPNs generally need about 1.0 to 1.5 grams of protein per kilogram of body weight per day. Protein requirements vary depending on the underlying disease state. A severely malnourished patient may require upto to 1.5 grams of protein per day, provided that the higher amount can safely be administered.

Sample Total Parenteral Nutrition

A sample TPN may have the following ingredients and quantities:

1)	Amino Acids	70 grams	Source: Travasol 10%
2)	Lipids	45 grams	Source: Liposyn® 20%
3)	Dextrose	385 grams	Source: Dextrose 50%
4)	Sodium Phosphate	27 mmol	Source: 3 mmol/ml
5)	Magnesium Sulfate	16 mEq	Source: 4.06 mEq/ml
6)	Calcium Gluconate	10 mEq	Source: 0.465 mEq/ml
7)	Potassium Acetate	140 mEq	Source: 4 mEq/ml
8)	Heparin	5000 units	Source: 5000 units/ml
9)	Ranitidine	300 mg	Source: 25 mg/ml
10)	Multivitamins	15 ml	Source: no concentration
11)	Trace Elements	7 ml	Source: no concentration
12)	Insulin	50 units	Source: 100 units/ml

Practice Problems: Calculate the volume of each ingredient needed.

1) Travasol 10% has 10 grams of amino acids in 100 ml and you need 70 grams. Write a proportion:

$$\frac{100 \text{ ml}}{10 \text{ grams}} = \frac{X \text{ ml}}{70 \text{ grams}}$$

X ml represents the volume of amino acid solution that has 70 grams of amino acids.

Isolate X ml by multiplying both sides by 70 grams:

$$\frac{70 \text{ grams} \times 100 \text{ ml}}{10 \text{ grams}} = \frac{X \text{ ml}}{\cancel{70 \text{ grams}}} \times \cancel{70 \text{ grams}}$$

This simplifies to:

$$\frac{70 \text{ grams} \times 100 \text{ ml}}{10 \text{ grams}} = X \text{ ml}$$

Divide 70 grams by 10 grams:

$$7 \times 100 \text{ ml} = X \text{ ml}$$

Finallly, $700 \text{ ml} = X \text{ ml}$

You need 700 ml of solution.

2)   Liposyn® 20% has 20 grams of lipids in 100 ml and you need 45 grams of lipids. Write a proportion as:

$$\frac{100 \text{ ml}}{20 \text{ grams}} = \frac{X \text{ ml}}{45 \text{ grams}}$$

Multiply both sides by 45 grams:

$$\frac{45 \text{ grams} \times 100 \text{ ml}}{20 \text{ grams}} = \frac{X \text{ ml}}{\cancel{45 \text{ grams}}} \times \cancel{45 \text{ grams}}$$

This simplifies to:

$$\frac{45 \text{ grams} \times 100 \text{ ml}}{20 \text{ grams}} = X \text{ ml}$$

Divide 45 grams by 20 grams:

$$2.25 \times 100 \text{ ml} = X \text{ ml}$$

Finally, $225 \text{ ml} = X \text{ ml}$

You need 225 ml of solution.

3)   The dose is 385 grams of dextrose and you have a solution of 50% dextrose. Write as proportion as:

$$\frac{100 \text{ ml}}{50 \text{ grams}} = \frac{X \text{ ml}}{385 \text{ grams}}$$

Multiply both sides by 385 grams:

$$\frac{385 \text{ grams} \times 100 \text{ ml}}{50 \text{ grams}} = \frac{X \text{ ml}}{385 \text{ grams}} \times 385 \text{ grams}$$

This simplifies to:

$$\frac{385 \text{ grams} \times 100 \text{ ml}}{50 \text{ grams}} = X \text{ ml}$$

Divide 385 grams by 50 grams:

$$7.7 \times 100 \text{ ml} = X \text{ ml}$$

Finally, $770 \text{ ml} = X \text{ ml}$

You need 770 ml of solution.

4)   You need 27 mmol of sodium phosphate based on the phosphate concentration not the sodium concentration. The phosphate concentration is 3 mmol/ml. Write as proportion as:

$$\frac{1 \text{ ml}}{3 \text{ mmol}} = \frac{X \text{ ml}}{27 \text{ mmol}}$$

Multiply both sides by 27 mmol:

$$\frac{27 \text{ mmol} \times 1 \text{ ml}}{3 \text{ mmol}} = \frac{X \text{ ml}}{27 \text{ mmol}} \times 27 \text{ mmol}$$

This simplifies to:

$$\frac{27 \text{ mmol} \times 1 \text{ ml}}{3 \text{ mmol}} = X \text{ ml}$$

Divide 27 mmol by 3 mmol:

$$9 \times 1 \text{ ml} = X \text{ ml}$$

Finally, $9 \text{ ml} = X \text{ ml}$

You need 9 ml of sodium phosphate.

5)   The dose is 16 mEq of magnesium sulfate and the concentration is 4.06 mEq/ml. Write a proportion as:

$$\frac{1 \text{ ml}}{4.06 \text{ mEq}} = \frac{X \text{ ml}}{16 \text{ mEq}}$$

Multiply both sides by 16 mEq:

$$\frac{16 \text{ mEq} \times 1 \text{ ml}}{4.06 \text{ mEq}} = \frac{X \text{ ml}}{16 \text{ mEq}} \times 16 \text{ mEq}$$

This simplifies to:

$$\frac{16 \text{ mEq} \times 1 \text{ ml}}{4.06 \text{ mEq}} = X \text{ ml}$$

Divide 16 mEq by 4.06 mEq:

$$3.94 \times 1 \text{ ml} = X \text{ ml}$$

Finally, $3.94 \text{ ml} = X \text{ ml}$

You need 3.94 ml of solution.

6)   The dose is 10 mEq of calcium gluconate and the concentration is 0.465 mEq/ml. Write a proportion as:

$$\frac{1 \text{ ml}}{0.465 \text{ mEq}} = \frac{X \text{ ml}}{10 \text{ mEq}}$$

Multiply both sides by 10 mEq:

$$\frac{10 \text{ mEq} \times 1 \text{ ml}}{0.465 \text{ mEq}} = \frac{X \text{ ml}}{10 \text{ mEq}} \times 10 \text{ mEq}$$

This simplifies to:

$$\frac{10 \text{ mEq} \times 1 \text{ ml}}{0.465 \text{ mEq}} = X \text{ ml}$$

Divide 10 mEq by 0.465 mEq:

$$21.5 \times 1 \text{ ml} = X \text{ ml}$$

Finally, $21.5 \text{ ml} = X \text{ ml}$

You need 21.5 ml of solution.

7)   The dose is 140 mEq of potassium acetate and the concentration is 4 mEq/ml. Write a proportion as:

$$\frac{1 \text{ ml}}{4 \text{ mEq}} = \frac{X \text{ ml}}{140 \text{ mEq}}$$

Multiply both sides by 140 mEq:

$$\frac{140 \text{ mEq} \times 1 \text{ ml}}{4 \text{ mEq}} = \frac{X \text{ ml}}{140 \text{ mEq}} \times 140 \text{ mEq}$$

This simplifies to:

$$\frac{140 \text{ mEq} \times 1 \text{ ml}}{4 \text{ mEq}} = X \text{ ml}$$

Divide 140 mEq by 4 mEq:

$$35 \times 1 \text{ ml} = X \text{ ml}$$

Finally, $35 \text{ ml} = X \text{ ml}$

You need 35 ml of solution.

8)   The dose is 5000 units of heparin and the concentration of the vial is 5000 units/ml. You need 1 ml of solution.

9)   The dose is 300 mg of ranitidine and the concentration is 25 mg/ml. Write a proportion as:

$$\frac{1 \text{ ml}}{25 \text{ mg}} = \frac{X \text{ ml}}{300 \text{ mg}}$$

Multiply both sides by 300 mg:

$$\frac{300 \text{ mg} \times 1 \text{ ml}}{25 \text{ mg}} = \frac{X \text{ ml}}{\cancel{300 \text{ mg}}} \times \cancel{300 \text{ mg}}$$

This simplifies to:

$$\frac{300 \text{ mg} \times 1 \text{ ml}}{25 \text{ mg}} = X \text{ ml}$$

Divide 300 mg by 25 mg:

$$12 \times 1 \text{ ml} = X \text{ ml}$$

Finally,　　　　　$12 \text{ ml} = X \text{ ml}$

You need 12 ml of solution.

10)　For multivitamins you simply measure out the same volume the doctor ordered and add it to the TPN.

11)　For trace elements you simply measure out the same volume the doctor ordered and add it to the TPN.

12)　The dose is 50 units and the concentration is 100 units/ml. Write a proportion as:

$$\frac{1 \text{ ml}}{100 \text{ units}} = \frac{X \text{ ml}}{50 \text{ units}}$$

Multiply both sides by 50 units:

$$\frac{50 \text{ units} \times 1 \text{ ml}}{100 \text{ units}} = \frac{X \text{ ml}}{\cancel{50 \text{ units}}} \times \cancel{50 \text{ units}}$$

This simplifies to:

$$\frac{50 \text{ units} \times 1 \text{ ml}}{100 \text{ units}} = X \text{ ml}$$

Divide 50 units by 100 units:

$$0.5 \times 1 \text{ ml} = X \text{ ml}$$

Finally, $0.5 \text{ ml} = X \text{ ml}$

You need 0.5 ml of insulin regular.

Review

Some patients are not able to physically eat or swallow liquids or may have limited ability to eat or swallow liquids. In these instances, patients will need enteral nutrition or parenteral nutrition. Enteral nutrition is preferred over parenteral nutrition because overall it has less risks, including decreased risk of systemic infection and no risk of venous blood clots. Some enteral products that have a high osmolality may need to be diluted with water based on a physicians instructions. Total parenteral nutrition is used as a last resort. It is a large volume IV that has amino acids, lipids, dextrose, vitamins, trace elements, heparin, insulin, and ranitidine. Specific ingredients and amounts vary depending on a particular patient's needs. TPNs may cause blood clots so heparin is used to prevent clotting. Insulin is added to maintain normal blood sugar levels. TPNs may be administered over a wide range of hours extending to a full 24 hours. You will be required to calculate the number of ml administered per hour so the IV pump can be set correctly.

Appendix

Practice Test #1

1)	A prescription is written for clarithromycin 500 mg tablets: take 1 tablet b.i.d. for 7 days. How many tablets does the patient need?

2)	Prescriptions are written for 1) enoxaprin 100 mg: inject 100 mg b.i.d. for 5 days, and 2) warfarin 5 mg once daily. How many mg of warfarin will the patient take in 5 days?

3)	A 1000 ml IV of normal saline is administered over 12 hours. What is the rate per hour?

4)	A 1000 ml IV of normal saline is administered over 10 hours. What is the rate per hour?

5)	A 1000 ml IV of normal saline is administered over 8 hours. What is the rate per hour?

6)	A 1000 ml IV of normal saline is administered over 5 hours. What is the rate per hour?

7)	A 1000 ml IV of normal saline is administered over 4 hours. What is the rate per hour?

8)	A 70 kg patient received a 70 mg per kg bolus dose of heparin. How many mg did the patient receive?

9)	A 80 kg patient received a 70 mg per kg bolus dose of heparin. How many mg did the patient receive?

10)	A 100 kg patient is receiving 18 mg per kg of heparin per hour. How many units of heparin does the patient receive each hour?

11)	A 100 kg patient is receiving 18 mg per kg of heparin per hour. How many units of heparin does the patient need in 12 hours?

12)	A prescription states: insulin regular sig: inject 10 units three times daily. How many units is the patient using every 30 days?

13)   A prescription states: insulin NPH sig: inject 20 units once daily. How many units is the patient using every 30 days?

14)   A medication order is written for 500 ml of 1/2 normal saline to be infused over 4 hours. A tubing is marked 15gtts per ml. What is the drip rate?

15)   A medication order is written for 1000 ml of normal saline to be infused over 8 hours. A tubing is marked 10 drops per ml. What is the drip rate?

16)   A prescription is written for amoxicillin 250 mg/5 ml. A patient is to receive 5 ml three times daily for 10 days. How many ml does the patient need for 10 days?

17)   An order is written for 950 mg of drug "A." The stock vial has a concentration of 20 mg/ml. How many ml are needed for the dose?

18)   A medication order is written for 500 mg of drug "B." The stock vial has a concentration of 50 mg/ml. How many ml are needed for the dose?

19)   A prescription is written for 100 mg of amantadine to be given twice daily. How many ml of the manufacturer's stock solution are needed for one dose if the concentration is 50 mg/5ml?

20)   A medication order is written for a 70 kg adult patient for IV allopurinol dosed at 200 mg/m^2 daily. The patient has a body surface area of 1.73 m^2. What is the dose?

21)   A stock vial of a drug has 10 ml of a 1% weight in volume solution. How many grams of drug are in the 10 ml?

22)   A medication order is written for allopurinol 1 mg/kg daily for a patient who weighs 100 kg. What is the dose?

23)   What is 0.45% in ratio strength?

24)   What is 0.55% in ratio strength?

25)   What is 0.35% in ratio strength?

26)   What is 1:1000 in percentage strength?

27)   What is 1:2000 in percentage strength?

28)   What is 1:3500 in percentage strength?

29)   What is 1:200 in percentage strength?

30)   What is 1:10,000 in percentage strength?

31)   A medication order reads 900 ml of normal saline (0.9%) to be administered over 6 hours. The IV tubing is marked 10 drops per 1 ml. What is the drip rate?

32)   A medication order reads 850 ml of normal saline to be administered over 5 hours. The IV tubing is marked 10 drops per 1 ml. What is the drip rate?

33)   A medication order reads 1000 ml of D5W to be administered over 7 hours. The tubing is marked 15 drops per 1 ml. What is the drip rate?

34)   A medication order reads 750 ml of normal saline to be administered over 5 hours. The IV tubing is marked 15 drops per 1 ml. What is the drip rate?

35)   A medication order reads 750 ml of normal saline to be administered over 5 hours. The tubing is marked 60 drops per 1 ml. What is the drip rate?

36)   A child has a BSA of 1.60 m^2. The adult dose of a drug is 175 mg. What is the child's dose based on BSA?

37)   A child has a BSA of 1.384 m^2. The adult dose of a drug is 200 mg. What is the child's dose based on BSA?

38)   A child has a BSA of 1.211 m². The adult dose of a drug is 100 mg. What is the child's dose based on BSA?

39)   A child has a BSA of 1.73 m². The adult dose of a drug is 75 mg. What is the child's dose based on BSA?

40)   A child has a BSA of 0.865 m². The adult dose of a drug is 200 mg. What is the child's dose based on BSA?

41)   A prescription is written for lactulose solution 10 g/15ml. How many grams of lactulose are in a 473 ml stock bottle?

42.   A doctor orders 900 units per hour of heparin. You have a pre-mixed IV bag of 25,000 units in 500 ml. How many ml per hour does the patient need?

43.   A doctor orders an IV bolus dose of 80 units per kilogram for a patient weighing 90 kilograms. You have a stock vial of 5000 units per 1 ml. How many ml are required for the dose?

44.   A medication order for ceftazidime 500 mg IM every 8 hours is written for an adult patient. How many mg are required for 24 hours of dosing?

45.   A medication order for ceftazidime 50 mg/kg every 8 hours is written for a patient weighing 50 kg. How many mg are needed for 24 hours of dosing.

46.   A medication order is written for ceftriaxone 2 grams every 12 hours for 14 days. What is the total dose the patient received after 14 days?

47.   A medication order was written for heparin 12 units/kg/hour for a patient weighing 83 kg. How many units will the patient receive in 24 hours?

48.   A medication order is written for an IV bolus dose of heparin 80 units/kg for a patient weighing 70 kg. A stock vial has 1000 units/ml.

How many ml are needed for the bolus dose?

49.   An 1000 ml IV has been running at a rate of 80 ml/hour for 3 hours. How many ml are left in the IV bag?

50.   A patient is receiving D5W at 100 ml/hour. How many grams of dextrose is the patient receiving each hour?

51.   A patient is receiving D5W at 80 ml/hour. The IV bag is 500 ml. How many grams of dextrose are in the IV bag?

52.   A prescription is written for dexamethasone 2 mg orally daily for three days. The pharmacy only has 0.25 mg tablets. How many tablets does the patient need for each dose?

53)   What is the drip rate for a 300 ml IV that is running over 4 hours provided the tubing is labeled 20 drops/ml?

54)   What is the drip rate for a 500 ml IV that is running over 4 hours provided the tubing is labeled 15 drops/ml?

55)   What is the drip rate for a 1000 ml IV that is running over 7 hours provided the tubing is labeled for 20 drops/ml?

56)   What is the drip rate for a 400 ml IV that is running over 7 hours provided the tubing is labeled 15 drops/ml?

57)   What is the drip rate for a 550 ml IV that is running over 5 hours provided the tubing is labeled 15 drops/ml?

58)   What is the drip rate for a 1000 ml IV that is running over 8 hours provided the tubing is labeled 10 drops/ml?

59)   A prescription is written for 150 grams of triamcinolone 0.1% cream mixed with cream base 1:1. How many grams of triamcinolone cream are needed?

60)   A prescription is written for 150 grams of triamcinolone 0.1%

mixed with cream base 1:1. How many grams of cream base are needed?

61)   A prescription is written for 150 grams of triamcinolone 0.1% mixed with cream base 1:2. How many grams of triamcinolone cream are needed?

62)   A prescription is written for 150 grams of triamcinolone 0.1% cream mixed with cream base 1:2. How many grams of cream base are needed?

63)   A patient is receiving a 2000 ml TPN over 24 hours. How many ml per hour is the patient receiving?

64)   A patient is receiving a 1500 ml TPN over 12 hours. What is the flow rate per hour?

65)   A patient is receiving a 2000 ml TPN over 24 hours that has 150 grams of lipids. How many grams of fat is the patient receiving each hour?

66)   A doctor orders 75 units of insulin regular three times daily. How many ml of insulin is the patient receiving every 24 hours?

67)   In the avoirdupois system, how many ounces equal one pound?

68)   How many ml are in one teaspoon?

69)   How many ml are in one tablespoon?

70)   How many grams are in one kilogram?

71)   How many milliliters are in one liter?

72)   How many mg are in 1000 mcg?

73)   One pound equals how many kg?

74)   One kg equals how many pounds?

75)   A medication order is written for 4.5 mg/kg of lidocaine. What is the dose for a patient weighing 70 kg?

76)   A medication order is written for 1.5 mg/kg of lidocaine. What is the dose for a patient weighing 100 kg?

77)   A medication order is written for 1 mg/kg of lidocaine for a patient weighing 75 kg. What is the dose?

78)   A prescription is written for 240 grams of hydrocortisone 1% cream mixed with cream base 1:3. How many grams of hydrocortisone are needed?

79)   A prescription is written for insulin glulisine 75 units once daily. How many ml are needed for this dose?

80)   A medication order is written for ondansetron 0.15 mg/kg three times daily for a patient weighing 220 pounds. A stock vial has 2 mg/ml. How many ml are needed for this dose?

81)   A medication order is written for ondansetron 0.45 mg/kg once daily. The patient weighs 190 pounds. A stock vial has 2 mg/ml. How many ml are needed for this dose?

82)   A medication order is written for oprelvekin 50 mcg/kg for a patient weighing 100 kg. How many mg does this patient need?

83)   A medication order is written for panitumumab 6 mg/kg for a patient weighing 90 kg. A 10 ml stock vial has 20 mg/ml. How many mg are in the stock bottle?

84)   A medication order is written for fluocinonide 0.05% ointment to be applied 4 times daily to the affected area. The pharmacy dispenses a 60 gram tube. How many grams of the active ingredient, fluocinonide, are in the tube?

85)   A doctor orders 1500 ml of normal saline over 8 hours. What rate will you set the pump at?

86)   A doctor orders 500 ml of D5W over 6 hours. The tubing set is labeled 20 drops per ml. What is the drip rate?

87)   A drug has a concentration of 0.1 grams in 100 ml. What is its ratio strength?

88)   A doctor orders ampicillin 75 mg/kg/day in divided doses every 6 hours for a patient weighing 50 kg. How many mg are in each dose?

89)   A patient is receiving lisinopril 30 mg tablets twice daily. The pharmacy only has 10 mg tablets. How many tablets per day is the patient using?

90)   A patient is receiving 1000 units of heparin per hour. The pharmacy sends a 100 ml IV bag with 10,000 units. How many hours will the IV bag last?

91)   A patient is receiving 1000 units of heparin per hour. The pharmacy sends a 100 ml IV bag with 10,000 units. How many ml per hour should the patient receive?

92)   A patient is receiving 1000 units of heparin per hour. The pharmacy sends a 1000 ml IV bag with 20,000 units. If the pharmacy used 4 ml from a stock vial, what was the concentration in the stock vial?

93)   A 10 ml stock vial has 1000 units of heparin per ml. How many 5000 units bolus doses of heparin can be prepared from this one stock vial?

94)   A 1000 ml IV of normal saline has been infused at 75 ml per hour for 10 hours. How many ml are left in the bag?

95)   A medication order is written for phenytoin sodium 100 mg every 8 hours. The stock vial has 50 mg/ml. How many ml are needed for 24 hours of dosing?

96)   A 40 kg patient is to receive 5 mg/kg of phenytoin daily in two divided doses. The stock vial has phenytoin sodium 50 mg/ml. How many ml are needed for one dose?

97)   A patient is receiving 600 mg daily of phenytoin oral suspension in 3 divided doses. You have a stock container of 125 mg/5 ml. How many ml are needed for one individual dose?

98)   A patient is receiving 600 mg daily of phenytoin oral suspension in 3 divided doses. You have a 240 ml stock container of 125 mg/5ml of phenytoin suspension. How many ml are needed for 24 hours of dosing?

99)   A medication order is written for a 15 mg/kg loading dose of phenytoin for a 100 kg patient. How many mg are needed for the loading dose?

100)   A medication order is written for IV sotalol 150 mg twice daily. The stock vial has 15 mg/ml. How many ml are needed for one dose?

Practice Test #2

1)   A 1000 ml IV bag of heparin with 36,000 units of heparin has been sent by the pharmacy to the nursing station for a patient. If the patient is receiving 1,500 units of heparin per hour, and the dose is 15 units/kg per hour, then what is the patient's weight in pounds?

2)   A 900 ml IV bag of heparin with 36,000 units of heparin has been sent by the pharmacy to the nursing station for a patient. If the bag lasts for 24 hours, then what was the drip rate for tubing labeled 60 drops/ml?

3)   A 70 kg patient is receiving 15 units/kg of heparin per hour for 24 hours. The IV bag has 1000 ml. Provided the IV bag has the correct amount of heparin for 24 hours, how many units of heparin are in each 1 ml of IV solution?

4)   A 70 kg patient is to receive 15 units/kg of heparin per hour for 24 hours. The IV bag has 1000 ml. Provided the IV bag has the correct amount of heparin for 24 hours, how many ml of heparin are needed from a stock vial that has 10,000 units per 2 ml?

5)   A 1000 ml IV bag of heparin with 20 units per ml has been running for 2 hours at 25 ml/hour. How many units of heparin has the patient received?

6)   A 500 ml IV bag of heparin with 18,000 units of heparin has been sent by the pharmacy to the nursing station for a patient. If the bag lasts for 24 hours, then what was the drip rate for tubing labeled 20 drops/ml?

7)   A 90 kg patient is receiving 900 units of heparin per hour. What is the dose per kg of body weight per hour?

8)   A 100 kg patient is receiving 1500 units of heparin per hour. What is the dose per kg of body weight per hour?

9)   A 100 kg patient has been receiving 12 units of heparin per kg per hour. If the IV bag had 14,400 units originally and now has 7,200 units, how many hours has the IV bag been infused?

10)   A 100 kg patient has been receiving 15 units of heparin per kg per hour for 12 hours. If the IV bag has 4500 units left, how many more hours can the bag be used?

11)   A prescription is written for insulin regular U-100 inject 40 units three times daily. How many units does the patient use in 30 days?

12)   A prescription is written for insulin regular U-100 inject 40 units three times daily. How many ml does the patient use in 30 days?

13)   Referring to question 12, how many 10 ml insulin vials will the patient need every 28 days?

14)   A prescription is written for 150 units of insulin regular U-500 to be injected twice daily. How many ml does the patient need per dose?

15)   A prescription is written for insulin NPH 20 units twice daily. How many units does the patient use in 28 days?

16)   A prescription is written for 10 units of insulin glargine to be injected once daily. Insulin glargine vials have 100 units per ml. How many ml does the patient need for one dose?

17)   A prescription is written for insulin glargine 30 units twice daily. The insulin glargine vial has 100 units per ml and 10 ml total. How many units are in one bottle?

18)   A prescription is written for insulin detemir 25 units once daily. At this dose, how many doses are in a 10 ml vial that has 100 units per ml?

19)   A prescription is written for insulin lispro 50 units three times daily. How many doses of 50 units each are in a 10 ml stock vial that has 100 units per ml?

20)   A prescription is written for 20 units of insulin aspart. How many doses are in a 10 ml stock vial that has 100 units per ml?

21)   What is 0.1% in ratio strength?

22)   What is 0.01% in ratio strength?

23)   What is 0.001% in ratio strength?

24)   What is 0.2% in ratio strength?

25)   What is 0.3 % in ratio strength?

26)   What is 1:100 in percentage strength?

27)   What is 1:200 in percentage strength?

28)   What is 1:1000 in percentage strength?

29)   What is 1:2000 in percentage strength?

30)   What is 1:3000 in percentage strength?

31)   A TPN needs 30 mmol of sodium phosphate. A stock vial has 3 mmol/ml. How many ml of the sodium phosphate stock vial are needed for the TPN?

32)   A TPN needs 20 mEQ of magnesium sulfate. A stock vial has 4.06 mEq/ml. How many ml are needed?

33)   A TPN needs 20 mEq of calcium gluconate. A stock vial has 0.465 mEq/ml. How many ml are needed?

34)   A 2000 ml TPN is being infused over 24 hours. How many ml per hour is the patient receiving?

35)   A 1000 ml TPN is being infused over 12 hours. How many ml per hour is the patient receiving?

36)   A 2000 ml TPN has 60 grams of lipids. You have a stock vial of lipids at 30%. How many ml of the stock vial are needed to supply 60 grams of lipids?

37)   A 1500 ml TPN has 50 grams of lipids. You have a stock vial of lipids 20%. How many ml of the stock vial are needed to supply 50 grams of lipids?

38)   A 2000 ml TPN has 80 grams of amino acids. A stock vial of amino acids has a concentration of 10%. How many ml of the stock vial are needed for the TPN?

39)   A TPN needs 400 grams of dextrose. You have three different strengths of dextrose: 10%, 50%, and 70%. Which one requires the

least volume for the 400 gram dose of dextrose?

40)   A child has a body surface area of 1.557 m². The adult dose of a drug is 100 mg. Using body surface area (BSA), what is the child's dose?

41)   A child has a body surface area of 1.384 m². The adult dose is 200 mg. Using body surface area (BSA), what is the child's dose?

42)   A child has a body surface area of 1.298 m². The adult dose is 300 mg. Using body surface area (BSA), what is the child's dose?

43)   A child has a body surface area of 1.211 m². The adult dose is 100 mg. Using body surface area (BSA), what is the child's dose?

44)   A child has a body surface area of 1.038 m². The adult dose is 120 mg. Using body surface area (BSA), what is the child's dose?

45)   A child has a body surface area of 1.73 m². The adult dose is 100 mg. Using body surface area (BSA), what is the child's dose?

46)   One kilogram equals how many pounds?

47)   One pound equals how many kilograms?

48)   How many ml are in one teaspoon?

49)   How many teaspoons are in 30 ml?

50)   How many ml are in one tablespoon?

51)   How many ml are in one liter?

52)   0.5 liter has how many ml?

53)   One kilogram has how many grams?

54)   One grain equals how many mg?

55) A pound (avoirdupois) has how many grams?

56) 1 fluid ounce equals how many ml?

57) A pint has how many ounces?

58) Convert 250 mg to grams.

59) Convert 500 mg to grams.

60) Convert 1.5 grams to mg.

61) Convert 1.5 liters to ml.

62) Convert 900 ml to liters.

63) Convert 220 pounds to kg.

64) Convert 100 kg to pounds.

65) One gallon has how many ml?

66) A patient is receiving 1500 ml of normal saline over 4 hours. How many ml per hour is the patient receiving?

67) A patient is receiving 2000 ml of normal saline over 8 hours. How many ml per hour is the patient receiving?

68) A patient is receiving 500 ml of 1/2 normal saline over 4 hours. How many ml per hour is the patient receiving?

69) A patient is receiving 750 ml of normal saline over 5 hours. How many ml per hour is the patient receiving?

70) A patient is receiving 1000 ml of 1/2 normal saline over 10 hours. How many ml per hour is the patient receiving?

71) A patient is receiving 1000 ml of D5W (dextrose 5% in water)

over 8 hours. How many ml of D5W is the patient receiving every hour?

72)   Referring to question 71, how many grams of dextrose is the patient receiving every hour?

73)   A patient is receiving 500 ml of D5W every 4 hours. Over a 4 hour interval, how many grams of dextrose does the patient receive?

74)   A patient is receiving 1000 ml of D5W every 12 hours. How many grams of dextrose is the patient receiving from the 1000 ml?

75)   A patient is receiving 2000 ml of D5W every 8 hours. How many grams of dextrose is the patient receiving from the 2000 ml?

76)   A patient is receiving 1000 ml of normal saline every 8 hours by IV drip. The tubing is marked 10 drops per ml. How many drops per minute is the patient receiving?

77)   A patient is receiving 500 ml of normal saline every 6 hours by IV drip. The tubing is marked 20 drops per ml. How many drops per minute is the patient receiving?

78)   A patient is receiving 2000 ml of 1/2 normal saline every 7 hours by IV drip. The tubing is marked 10 drops per ml. How many drops per minute is the patient receiving?

79)   A patient is receiving 750 ml of 1/2 normal saline every 4 hours by IV drip. The tubing is marked 20 drops per ml. How many drops per minute is the patient receiving?

80)   A patient is receiving 850 ml of 1/2 normal saline every 3 hours by IV drip. The tubing is marked 10 drops per ml. How many drops per minute is the patient receiving?

81)   A doctor writes a medication order for gentamicin for 2.0 mg/kg per dose for a patient weighing 100 kg. The patient receives three doses daily. How many mg does a patient receive in 24 hours?

82)   Referring to the previous question, what would be the dose in terms of mg/kg if the patient received the entire days dose during one infusion?

83)   A doctor writes a medication order for gentamicin 5 mg/kg for a patient weighing 100 kg. You have a stock vial of 40 mg/ml. How many ml are needed for the dose?

84)   A doctor writes a medication order for gentamicin 1.5 mg/kg every 8 hours for a patient weighing 100 kg. You have a stock vial of 40 mg/ml. How many ml are needed for the dose?

85)   A doctor writes an order for gentamicin 8 mg per day to be injected intrathecally. You have a stock vial of 40 mg/ml. How many ml are needed for the dose?

86)   A medication order is written for dopamine 1 mcg/kg/minute. For a 100 kg patient, how many mg will be infused over 1 hour?

87)   A medication order is written for dopamine 5 mcg/kg/minute. For a 100 kg patient, how many mcg will be infused over 1 hour?

88)   A medication order is written for dopamine 20 mcg/kg/minute. For a 100 kg patient, how many mg will be infused over 1 hour?

89)   A medication order is written for dopamine 10 mcg/kg/minute for a 100 kg patient. A premixed IV bag with a concentration of 0.8 mg/ml is available. How many ml will the patient need every minute?

90)   A medication order is written for dopamine 5 mcg/kg per minute for a patient weighing 100 kg. You have a premixed IV bag with 1.6 mg/ml. How many ml will the patient need every hour?

91)   A prescription is written for amoxicillin 875 mg tablets every 8 hours for 10 days. How many tablets does the patient need for all ten days?

92)   A prescription is written for gemfibrozil 600 mg twice daily.

How many tablets will the patient need for 90 days?

93)   A prescription is written for atenolol 50 three times daily. How many tablets will the patient need for 90 days?

94)   A prescription is written for amoxicillin 250 mg/5ml to give 5 ml three times daily for 10 days. How many ml will the patient need for 10 days?

95)   A prescription is written for lisinopril 10 mg twice daily for 30 days. How many tablets will the patient need?

96)   A prescription is written for albuterol inhalation two puffs twice daily. An inhaler has 200 puffs total. How many days will one inhaler last?

97)   A prescription is written for albuterol inhalation two puffs four times daily. An inhaler has 200 puffs total. How many days will one inhaler last?

98)   A prescription is written for fluticasone nasal 1 puff twice daily in each nostril. One container has 120 puffs. How many days will one container last?

99)   A prescription is written for pirbuterol 2 inhalations every 6 hours. One inhaler has 400 puffs. How many days will one inhaler last?

100)   A teaspoon has how many ml?

Answers to Practice Test #1

1.   14
2.   25
3.   83.3 ml/hour
4.   100 ml/hour
5.   125 ml/hour

6.   200 ml/hour
7.   250 ml/hour
8.   4900 mg
9.   5600 mg
10.   1800 units/hour
11.   21,600 units
12.   900 units
13.   600 units
14.   31 drops/minute
15.   21 drops/minute
16.   150 ml
17.   47.5 ml
18.   10 ml
19.   10 ml
20.   346 mg
21.   0.1 grams
22.   100 mg
23.   1:222
24.   1:182
25.   1:286
26.   0.1%
27.   0.05%
28.   0.029%
29.   0.5%
30.   0.01%
31.   25 drops/minute
32.   28 drops/minute
33.   36 drops/minute
34.   38 drops/minute
35.   150 drops/minute
36.   161.8 mg
37.   160 mg
38.   70 mg
39.   75 mg
40.   100 mg
41.   315.3 grams
42.   18 ml/hour
43.   1.44 ml

44.   1500 mg
45.   7,500 mg
46.   56 grams
47.   23,904 units
48.   5.6 ml
49.   760 ml
50.   5 grams
51.   25 grams
52.   8 tablets
53.   25 drops/minute
54.   31 drops/minute
55.   48 drops/minute
56.   14 drops/minute
57.   28 drops/minute
58.   21 drops/minute
59.   75 grams
60.   75 grams
61.   50 grams
62.   100 grams
63.   83.3 ml/hour
64.   125 ml/hour
65.   6.25 grams/hour
66.   2.25 ml/24 hours
67.   16
68.   5 ml
69.   15 ml
70.   1000
71.   1000
72.   1
73.   0.454
74.   2.2
75.   315 mg
76.   150 mg
77.   75 mg
78.   60 grams
79.   0.75 ml
80.   7.5 ml
81.   19.4 ml

Page 144

82.   5 mg
83.   200 mg
84.   0.03 grams
85.   188 ml/hour
86.   28 drops/minute
87.   1:1000
88.   937.5 mg
89.   6
90.   10 hours
91.   10 ml
92.   5000 units/ml
93.   2
94.   250 ml
95.   6 ml
96.   2 ml
97.   8 ml
98.   24 ml
99.   1500 mg
100.   10 ml

Answers to Practice Test #2

1.   220 pounds
2.   38 drops/min
3.   25.2 units/ml
4.   5.04 ml
5.   1000 units
6.   7 drops/minute
7.   10 units/kg per hour
8.   15 units/kg per hour
9.   6 hours
10.   3 hours
11.   3,600 units
12.   36 ml
13.   4 vials
14.   0.3 ml
15.   1,120 units

16. 0.1 ml
17. 1000 units
18. 40 doses
19. 20 doses
20. 50 doses
21. 1:1000
22. 1:10,000
23. 1:100,000
24. 1:500
25. 1:333
26. 1%
27. 0.5%
28. 0.1%
29. 0.05%
30. 0.03%
31. 10 ml
32. 4.93 ml
33. 43 ml
34. 83.3 ml/hour
35. 83.3 ml/hour
36. 200 ml
37. 250 ml
38. 800 ml
39. 70%
40. 90 mg
41. 160 mg
42. 225 mg
43. 70 mg
44. 72 mg
45. 100 mg
46. 2.2 pounds
47. 0.454 kg
48. 5 ml
49. 6 teaspoons
50. 15
51. 1000
52. 500
53. 1000

54.   65 mg
55.   454 grams (also 480 grams)
56.   29.57 ml (also 30 ml)
57.   16 ounces
58.   0.250 grams
59.   0.5 grams
60.   1500 mg
61.   1500 ml
62.   0.9 liters
63.   100 kg
64.   220 pounds
65.   3785 ml
66.   375 ml/hour
67.   250 ml/hour
68.   125 ml/hour
69.   150 ml/hour
70.   100 ml/hour
71.   125 ml/hour
72.   6.25 grams/hour
73.   25 grams
74.   50 grams
75.   100 grams
76.   21 drops/minute
77.   28 drops/minute
78.   48 drops/minute
79.   63 drops/minute
80.   47 drops/minute
81.   600 mg
82.   6 mg/kg
83.   12.5 ml
84.   3.75 ml
85.   0.2 ml
86.   6 mg
87.   30,000
88.   120 mg
89.   1.25 ml/minute
90.   18.75 ml/hour
91.   30 tablets

92.	180 tablets
93.	270 tablets
94.	150 ml
95.	60 tablets
96.	50 days
97.	25 days
98.	30 days
99.	50 days
100.	5 ml.

Index

Printed in Great Britain
by Amazon